The REALLY SIMPLE diet:

Weight Loss that works!

A short guide to losing fat, getting healthier and feeling more energetic.

Max Bonpain

Founder of Back on Track

REVISED EDITION

Copyright © 2021 by MAX BONPAIN and BACK ON TRACK

Original Version first published in 2017

ISBN: 9798703511619

Table of Contents:

My story:

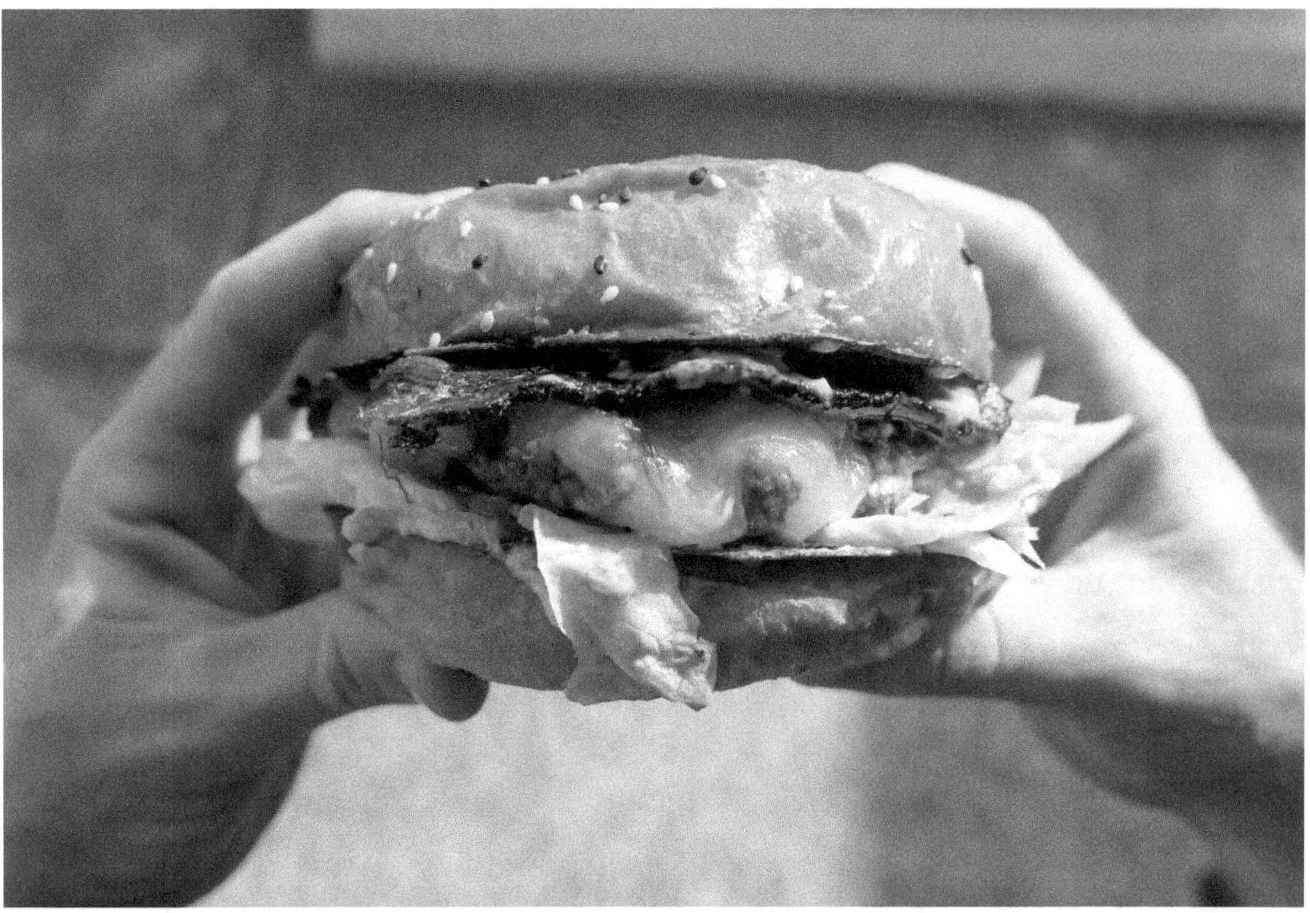

Now in my late 40s, I've been struggling with my weight for the last 20 years: naturally tall but not very muscular, I was quite thin until my 30s, when I started to put weight on. A couple of kilos per year, but soon I was over my ideal weight by 13 kilos and trying to get back on track.

I did what most people do in that case: I tried to do more sport and eat healthier, and through sheer will power, I managed –painfully- to get back to my ideal weight. However in my late 30s I started to put the weight back on, getting to my heaviest ever. I thought "well, I've managed to lose it once, I 'll be able to do it again the same way"… but no!

With the stubborn fat not melting away as hoped, I turned to diet books, full of hope and confidence. I was sorely disappointed: I tried a couple of low-carb diets, managed to "lose" a couple of kilos quite quickly, but put them back as quickly again, with a vengeance!

So I tried different diets, moving from low-carb to paleo, to keto and many others…. Over the years, I've tried many of the most popular diets without much success. I thought maybe it's my "macro" or my metabolism, and looked at other so-called "personalized" diet based on my DNA and other expensive tests: Nothing!

Desperate, I even tried supplements such as carb-blockers, meal replacements, matcha tea, metabolic boosters and sauna vests, wasting my money and my time.

Sounds familiar? Well, there is hope!

In the end, a couple of years ago, I decided to stop my scattergun approach and take a more scientific approach instead: As I was confused by the conflicting advices from one diet to the other, I decided to compare the "do / do not" from all the main diets out there and see what they agree on, assuming that the common part would be valid for most of us.

From there, I managed to draft list of a few principles (or rules, as you prefer) to follow, that helped me lose weight slowly but consistently (about half a kilo to a kilo per week), eventually reaching my target weight and staying there. To put it back in context, a kilo per week means 4 kilos per month so if you need to lose 30 kilos, at that pace it would take you about 8 months....

Let's be clear: there is no magic recipe or silver bullet that will get you to drop weight much faster than that (apart from medical procedures). Yes, you'll drop a couple of kilos in 24-48 hours on a no-carb diet, but that's because carbs retain water and when you stop carbs you lose that water (and the weight).

However that's not fat you've lost, and the water will be retained back as soon as you eat some carbs again... In my opinion, it's only "useful" if you need to drop a size to fit in a garment for a specific occasion or need to "make weight" for a MMA fight! But the benefit of a consistent weight loss is that, by definition, it's sustainable.

So, what is this short guide about?

This short guide is here to help you live a healthier life. Much of the information you need is freely available but confusing and often contradictory; we aim to simplify and give you clear guidelines that you can follow easily. But also you might simply not be aware of some of the recent learnings; we aim to inform you so you can decide based on facts.

In other words, why read 50 books when you can learn the most important facts from this one short guide?

Now, what do we mean by healthier life?

Our first tips will be about losing weight. However, although weight loss is usually helping for some weight-related conditions such as cholesterol, you can lose weight whilst following a nutrient-poor diet.

So, beyond the weight loss principles, we review what we learnt from all the diets out there that can help you feel better in mind and body, get your lifestyle and health under control thanks to simple guidelines, and get back on track. Yes, you will lose weight, but the right type of weight loss: Body fat, not water or muscle mass. Your mood will be lifted and you should be feeling better.

Why do I need this guide for this?

Well, if you read just one book about health, diet or nutrition, you might feel clear enough, although overwhelmed, about what to do next. But if you happen to read a second, let alone 3rd, 4th, and so on, book, chances are you'll be confused! It's because nutrition is complex and it's impossible to reconcile all points of view when they seem contradictory. In the end, bear in mind it's all about balance: there's no magic recipe, no secret ingredient, and no perfect food or diet. Whatever food you look into, you'll find pros and cons: miracle for some, evil for others, because food is chemically complex.

So, what to make about it? We'll choose the foods that have a positive balance: mostly good for you, and avoid the foods that have a negative balance, mostly bad for you. The better the food, the more we'll have. But bear in mind, nothing's perfect and the chemical complexity of food means that some diets will say "go for it" whilst others will say "no way" for the same food!

Examples abound: coffee, nuts, nightshade vegetables, broccoli, or even quinoa… All supposedly healthy foods (and foods we'll recommend) but that can have negative aspects as well: caffeine can increase cortisol (the stress hormone), nuts need to be soaked, quinoa and spinach contain oxalates, etc.

So: good or bad? In or out? Don't worry, we'll take you by the hand and help you make the best choices.

Why listen to me?

I'm not a physician, GP (General Practitioner, also known as MD, Medical Doctor) or a clinical nutritionist. But I've been through the same struggles and learnt the hard way. Most importantly, I've done the homework and I don't have any vested interest in any specific diet.

Beyond my weight-loss, I also gained an interest in nutrition. I'm someone who struggled with health issues for years, saw many different health professionals, including ENTs, nutritionists, gastros, endocrinos, which drove me to research the link between food and health, particularly energy (both physical and mental).

I did a series of tests, such as food allergies and organic acids: I found out that I am sensitive to cow's milk as well as wheat, have with a methylation problem with vitamin B12 and an excess of yeast (candida). No wonder why I had been feeling tired, almost lethargic most of my life!

So, this guide is my way to give back, to share my experience and what I learnt.

I'm not going through the theory – I've included a list of references if you want to understand the science. My aim is to give you a short cut to help you get back on track. I found that most "methods" have hundreds of pages for just a couple of big ideas. And usually they have a bunch of recipes using exotic ingredients only available in health shops that nobody prepares!

So this guide is to put all these big ideas in one place. And as you'll see, when you strip off the tinsel, the ideas are often not much more than common sense.

1 – Weight loss demystified

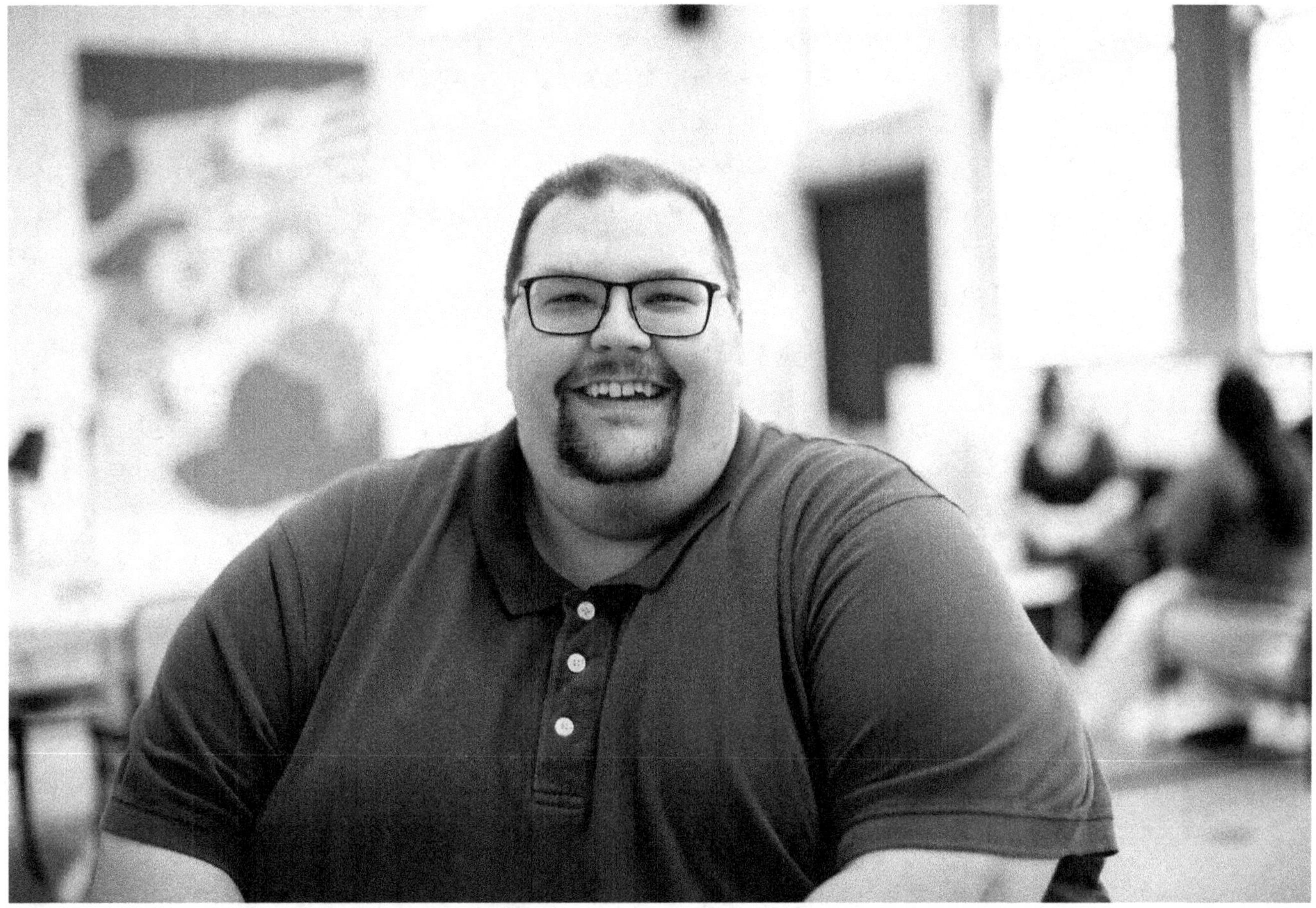

Let's cut to the chase: **there is only ONE way to lose weight**, and it's calorie control: in other words, ingest fewer calories than you burn. Yes, Weight Watchers DOES work, as long as you follow it and don't snack in between ;-)

Now when I talk to people, I hear a lot of counter-arguments:

-if it was that easy, nobody would be fat

-if that was true, why all these new diets?

Let's be clear, calorie control is NOT easy, that's why people are looking for "magical" diets that require no will-power and maybe even suggest a few magical ingredients.

So, weight loss is simple as a concept but hard to do because of the demand on will power. Let's see how to make it easier to follow, so you can get the results you want.

Firstly, you need to track your weight and –importantly- you body fat percentage; for this we recommend buying a smart scale. I personally use the Fitbit's Aria scale, linked to my Fitbit app. For men, a healthy body-fat level is 15-25% of total weight, whilst for women it is 20-30%. However you need to be on the lower end to look slim enough, and even lower to show off your abs!

On this, let's clarify a key point: to lose weight without changing your diet would require a LOT of physical activity.

My personal philosophy is that diet is the best way to lose weight, whilst exercise helps with toning the body, making it firmer. Both together, diet and exercise will help you feel more energised and are needed for good health.

Secondly, you need to track the calories you ingest; for this, you can download a free calorie-tracking app. I use MyFitnessPal (the free version). It's amazing how having to input what you eat makes you realize how much you're eating and which foods are adding most to your waistline. Quite often, you can make a few simple changes when you realize that "healthy" foods are not that good.

For instance, adding tomato sauce to minced meat or pasta can easily add a couple hundred calories to the dish… In other words, by being more conscious about what you are eating, you'll be able to make small changes to your daily routine, that hopefully will add up. For me for instance, I know that my daily latte (coffee with a lot of milk) is not a great choice. I'll still have it some days, but will try not to have it every day (or several times a day!) and have tea or black coffee instead, or better still, a glass of kombucha.

Note that in this section we're focused on calorie counting and weight loss, so the discussion about whether there are good and bad calories is for a later part of this guide. The idea is to take it step by step, so that the plan is manageable. Once you've found your weight loss routine, you can go further and try a specific diet for improved health.

Thirdly, you need to compute your metabolic rate (how many calories you burn per day when just resting) and the daily caloric intake that would be required for an average day. You can google it and find many free sites to calculate it. This depends on age, height, gender and activity level but the average for men is 2000-3000 calories and for women 1600-2400 calories.

Then you can set your weight-loss caloric goal, usually about 500 calories under your daily requirement, so you can lose weight consistently. As an example, I've set myself a goal of 1720 calories per day (vs 2300 requirements). At 500 calories of "deficit", for my height and activity level, that translates into losing about 100-150 grams per day, or up to 1 kilo per week (4 kilos per months).

You can lose weight faster by lowering even further your caloric goal, but it could have health implications, so please discussion with your physician first.

Note also that your weight loss doesn't follow the same pace all the time and will usually plateau (stabilize) after a while. At that stage, you'll need to take a close look at the macros (fats, carbs and proteins) as it's likely you'll need to increase protein levels if you want to keep losing fat.

Fourthly, if you can afford it, also invest in a Fitbit or Garmin tracker to track your steps, heart rate, sleep quality and other health measures. It will help you get an overview of your progress.

Getting started:
At this early stage, to get started, focus on calories rather than the food quality (we'll see that later): if you need a treat, treat yourself, but look at the calories and maybe reduce the amount eaten. In my case, I love chocolate but felt guilty about it: I tried to stop, but ended binging on other things and made it worse! Once I realized that, I switched back to having some (dark) chocolate, but making sure I don't over-do it!

The goal is to replace progressively what you have been eating by lower calorie, higher nutrition foods. But in the very short term, focus on one thing, the calories you are getting from the food and drinks you are putting in your mouth. It's likely you'll need to reduce or replace some of the usual suspects: high sugar and high fat foods such as sugary drinks, sauces, sugary cereals, Danish and pastries…
Amazingly, it's often just a couple of bad habits that make the difference between putting or losing weight…

Later on, we'll switch the focus to the quality of the food, once you've taken the habit of calorie counting and have started your weight loss journey. For instance, we'll discuss the difference between good and bad fats. For now, we'll treat all fats the same way, as a source of calories to be restricted.

You're obviously welcome to try and start with both quantity and quality in mind, but in my experience it makes the diet harder to follow. Please bear in mind that by reducing your calories and starting your weight loss, you've done a significant first step.

A few FAQs:

-Should I weigh myself daily?
No. Weekly is better. For the simple reason that most of the daily weight fluctuations is due to water loss / retention. You can lose or put on up to one kg in 24 hours pending what you eat, which could hide the fat loss. Weigh yourself weekly, and check both your total weight and you body fat %; they should both be going down. If your weight is going down but not your body fat %, that means you're potentially losing muscle mass as well and might need to increase your protein intake. If your weight is not going down in spite of your efforts, that might simply mean you're not taking ALL calories into account, for instance sauces added to dishes, snacks, milk in coffee…

-Should I take weight loss supplements?
Probably not: they usually don't hurt, but they also usually don't help much… and they can be really expensive! For instance, all these "metabolic boosters" do increase your metabolism, but only so slightly and therefore don't really make a big difference to your weight loss. Look at anything "filling" instead, ie high in fibers, or potentially meal replacements, assuming you have them instead of -and not in addition to- your meals. Don't have them long-term, maybe a couple of weeks to kick start your diet with something easy to prepare and keep with you.
Note we'll speak about vitamins and other health supplements later, which are a different story to weight loss ones.
By the way, forget about the "sweat vests": any weight loss would be due to water loss, not fat…

-Don't the other diets work? They might work in the short term, mostly because they restrict what you can eat (and therefore your caloric intake) and get rid of most of the weight gain culprits.
However for many people it's hard to stick long-term to these diets if they are not enjoyed and followed to the letter. You might love a big juicy steak and eggs and bacon, and therefore think a paleo or keto diet is perfect for you, but are they really healthy in the long-term if you overdo it? You still need your greens!
The advantage of the caloric restriction approach is that you proceed by small tweaks, so it's a healthier, leaner approach to your current diet – no fancy recipe or exotic ingredient, just a bit less high-caloric foods daily…
Note the diet recommendations we suggest later on focus on health, longevity and energy.

2 – Beyond weight-loss and towards an approach to a healthier lifestyle

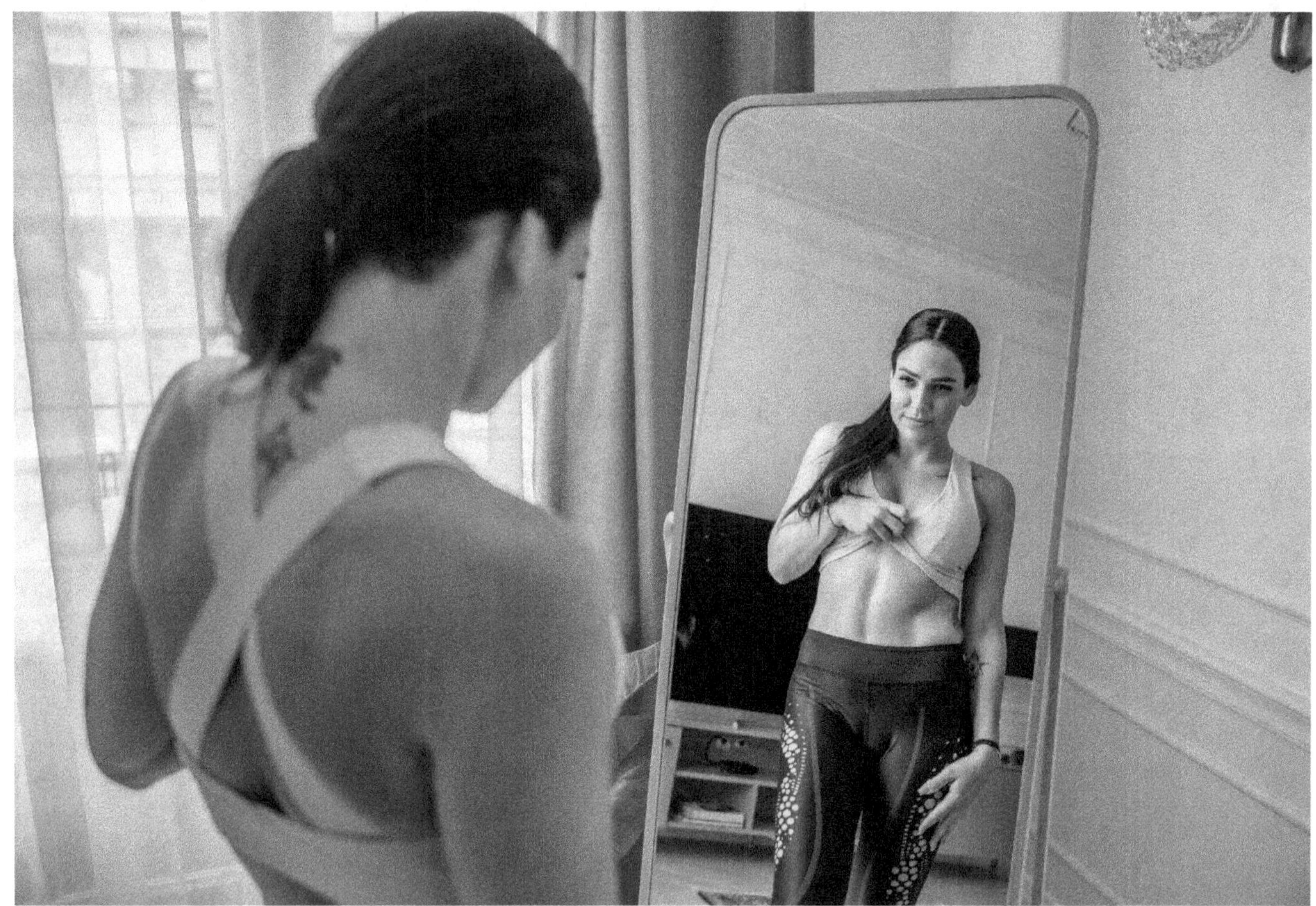

If you have any serious disease, such as diabetes or cholesterol, you quite likely know about it and already take some medication for it.

However your health, physical and mental, is not just defined by medical conditions and the associated medications prescribed; it's a lot more. You might just be feeling tired, have some skin rash, constipation, or any other of those "little things" that can make life miserable but are hard to diagnose and even harder to treat with medications. These require a change in lifestyle, but how do you know what changes to make?

If you've followed our advice from the previous section, you've started to lose weight and have found a routine that works for you, so what now? Well now we're going to get more specific about eating for health, not just weight.

As mentioned earlier, there are hundreds of competing diets out there. Which ones work? More importantly, which ones work for you specifically, if any?

If you're anything like me, you've probably tried a few diets already. Did that work for you? Well, most people lose some weight on a diet… and then put it back on and more! And I guess that's why you're reading this guide.

For that broader aim, here is the approach we'll follow:

-Firstly, we'll ask you to do a few tests to understand what can cause any condition ruining your health and life. These should be done under medical supervision – please discuss the results with your physician.

-Secondly, we'll take a step-by-step approach, rather than a one-size-fits-all, to help you find the best diet and lifestyle for you.

     Always consult a physician before starting a diet

Let's get your starting point: here is a list of symptoms, please check those you are currently experiencing.

*Please tick the box to the right of any condition you are **CURRENTLY EXPERIENCING**.*

GENERAL		WEIGHT		NERVOUS SYSTEM		EYES		EARS	
Fatigue		Weight gain		Headaches		Watery/itchy		Itchy	
Apathy/lethargy		Difficulty losing weight		Migraines		Painful/red		Ear aches	
Hyperactivity		Fluid retention		Faintness		Sticky eyelids		Infections	
Poor appetite		Binge eating		Dizziness		Blurred vision		Discharge	
Hypoglycaemia		Compulsive eating		Numbness		Deteriorating vision		Tinnitus (ringing)	
Poor sleep/insomnia		Craving for certain foods		Tingling, pins & needles		Dry eyes		Hearing loss	
Sleep apnoea		Weight loss		Poor co-ordination					
Excessive thirst		Eating disorders		Feel cold easily					
Stress				Cold hands & feet					
Easy bruising									

DIGESTIVE SYSTEM		HEART/CIRCULATION		LUNGS		GYNAECOLOGICAL		GENITO-URINARY	
Indigestion		High blood pressure		Shortness of breath		PMT (pre-menstrual syndrome)		Frequent urination	
Heartburn/reflux		Low blood pressure		Cough		Breast pain		Passing large amounts of urine	
Bloating		High cholesterol		Sputum		Breast lumps		Burning / discomfort on urination	
Feel full easily		Chest pain		Blood		Breast implants		Discharge	
Burping		Palpitations/arrhythmia		Chest tightness		Regular periods		Blood in urine	
Flatulence		Swelling of ankles		Wheeze		Irregular periods		Urgent urination	
Abdominal/stomach pains or cramps		Poor circulation				No periods		Kidney pain	
Nausea		Calf pain with exercise				Heavy periods		Difficulty passing urine	
Vomiting		Varicose veins				Menstrual clots		Passing urine frequently at night	
Difficulty swallowingxxxxxxx						Period pain/cramps		Incontinence	
Diarrhoea						Painful intercourse		Loss of libido	

Constipation					Vaginal irritation/soreness		Erectile dysfunction (impotence)	
Piles (haemorrhoids)					Vaginal discharge			
Mucus					Thrush			
Rectal bleeding					Menopausal			
Anal itching					Hot flushes			
					Sweats			
					Vaginal dryness			

NOSE		MOUTH / THROAT		SKIN		HAIR / NAILS		JOINTS / MUSCLES	
Congested/blocked		Mouth ulcers		Acne/pimples		HAIR		Pain	
Poor sense of smell		Cold sores		Eczema/dermatitis		Dry Hair		Swelling	
Sinus problems		Cracks at corner of mouth		Psoriasis		Increased hair loss		Stiffness	
Hay fever/allergy		Sore throat		Rosacea				Arthritis	
Sneezing		Hoarseness, loss of voice		Rashes		NAILS		Neck problems	
Excessive mucus		Gum disease/bleeding		Hives/urticaria		Soft		Back problems	
Post-nasal drip		Feeling of lump in throat		Dry skin		Break easily		Cramps / spasms	
		Loss of taste sensation		Poor healing		White spots		Muscle twitching	
		Bad breath		Excessive sweating		Ridged		Muscle tension	
				Body odour		Fungal infections		Muscle weakness	
				Dandruff				Gout	

EMOTIONS		MIND	
Anxiety		Poor memory	
Depression		Poor concentration	
Mood swings		Confusion	
Panic attacks		Poor comprehension	
Anger, irritability		'Brain fog'	

This will be your baseline. Please come back to this check-list every 3 months to check any improvement.

    Always consult a physician before starting a diet

<u>Testing</u>

First of all, you need to understand if anything is wrong with your health such as poor methylation, sleep apnea, poor digestion, hormones, etc.

I'd suggest seeing a specialist of integrative medicine (also known as functional medicine) and do a series of tests, including amino acids (OAT), food intolerance, toxins and even genetic testing (eg DNAFit).

If you are simply curious, there are quite a few tests you can do without a physician referral, but they won't be reimbursed by your health fund and might be difficult to interpret.

From the US, but available worldwide, Great Plains Laboratory does everything you need, including OAT. https://www.greatplainslaboratory.com/organic-acids-test/

You could also do genetic testing, especially for methylation issues: knowyourgenetics.com, or DNAFit.com provide these tests and give personalized recommendations. Genetics testing is quite new but very important: digestion is a chemical process, and the foods we eat alter our genes by switching them on and off – it's called epigenetics.

You would inherit your genes from your family, so look out for any disease your relatives suffer from as you are more likely to have these genes as well; however your lifestyle will influence to some extent whether they are switched on or off, in other words whether you are affected as well or not.

Your physician will advise for anything more specialized.

Overall, I'd suggest to only do the tests based to check for specific symptoms, rather than do everything. However one test I'd recommend to everybody is about food allergies and sensitivities, as they can be responsible for a bunch of symptoms, such as tiredness, reflux / GERD, IBS, and other digestive complications. You can do at your local allergy specialist for skin prick test, or through Great Plain Labs.

I'm not speaking about the "serious" (life-threatening) allergies, such as peanuts, but the ones that can make your life miserable without even realizing you are sensitive: the most common ones will be dairy (especially from cow's milk) and gluten/wheat. We'll cover allergens in detail later on.

<u>So here are the steps we will follow:</u>

1. Start to detox

2. Get your diet back under control

3. Focus on your sleep

4. Try and get some exercise back into your daily routine

5. Enjoy!

I speak about steps because you should not try and do everything at once: when you detox, you actually feel worse before you start feeling better. That's because all the toxins stored in your body (mainly in body fat) are released and go back through your system. During that time, you want to eat enough (good foods obviously), sleep as much as you can, and not exert yourself too much.

From that basis, you can move on to improving your diet; however it requires willpower and you should focus on one thing at the time. If exercise is your thing and makes you forget about the dieting effort, great. But if exercise is new for you, then better wait until you diet is under control.

Here is a timeline in weeks of the approach you could be taking

week 1	week 2	week 3	week 4	week 5	week 6	week 7	week 8	week 9	week 10	week 11	week 12
Follow the Better Sleep Guidelines											
Start meditation											
Start stretching and lunchtime walk					Add some light exercise, mixing cardio, HIIT and some weights						
		Detox									
				Diet Kickstart							
					Low carb, DF GF						
								Low Carb			
											Mediterranean

3 – Detox

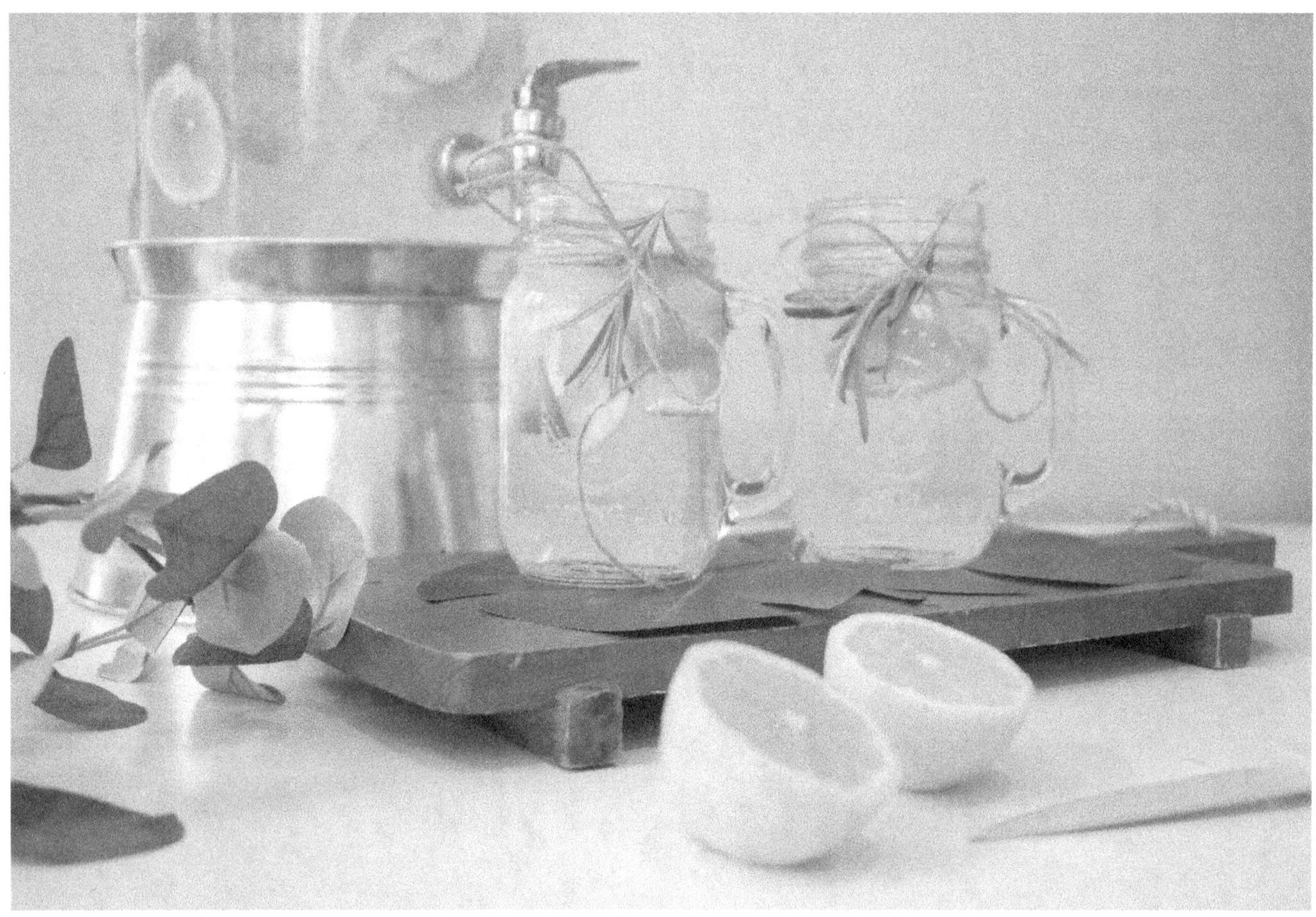

<u>Understanding your current toxic load</u>

To start with, we need to make sure you're not harming yourself unknowingly through food or environment.

We'll cover food in more detail later on, but you can also get toxins in your body through the air you breath (pollution) and the products you use: frying pans, plastic containers and bottles, skin or hair care products….

So, invest in a good air purifier and a water filter, vacuum your home and wash your bedding weekly, replace your non-stick cooking utensils by iron ones, check that all plastic food and drink containers are BPA-free and that all cosmetics are at least phthalates and parabens-free. The reason is that your skin absorbs the chemical from the products it comes in contact with.

It doesn't mean you should stop dying your hair or looking after yourself, just that you need to see if you can find an alternative product to the one you are currently using, so as to reduce the overall toxic load getting in your body one way or another.

          Always consult a physician before starting a diet

But let's be realistic, it's impossible to completely eliminate all toxins from the environment; we just want to try and avoid the main culprits, and compensate through a healthier lifestyle. Check www.cosmeticdatabase.com for detail. At home and in the office, get a few plants; they naturally detoxify the environment.

Regarding foods, have tuna no more than once a week due to mercury, and avoid pesticides / herbicides by buying organic whenever possible and washing your fruits and vegetables. Note we recommend washing rather than peeling as most of the nutrients are usually in the skin. Also, choose grass-fed, organic meat, to avoid added hormones and antibiotics.

But let's be clear, better have non-organic vegetables than no vegetables! If you can't afford organic, don't stress it too much.

All these toxins get stored in fat cells, so as not to overload the kidneys, and then get released back in the bloodstream when you detox or lose weight. So when you do, it's important to have anti-oxidants to bind with these toxins and take them out of your body, lest they get reabsorbed.

<u>Do I even need to detox?</u>

What are the telltale signs that you could benefit from a detox:

1 – low energy: you feel tired all the time.

2 – your skin, hair and nails: maybe you have dandruff or a rash, brittle nails, dry hair.

3 – your tongue: should not have any white or yellow coating, which are signs of candida (yeast infection, due to sugars being poorly digested).

4 – your stools: should be compact but not hard, with a brownish colour, and should not hurt.

5 – poor mood: feeling down, maybe depressed, often stressed.

If you are worried about anything, please go see a physician and discuss what you've found.

But detoxing your body, stopping sugar and some foods you might be sensitive to, sleeping better and exercising should bring you back on track.

There are extreme forms of detox, such as juicing, where you do not eat anything but green juices for a few days. Juicing is great because the nutrients go straight into your blood stream; however it should not be the only source of nutrition as the sugar also goes straight into your blood stream and it lacks fibre and other key nutrients. So juicing is great, but as a complement to your diet; see it as a boost. My favourite is a green juice with spinach, kale and watercress. Add pineapple or papaya to sweeten the taste and add digestive enzymes.

Sweating and drinking a lot will also help evacuate the toxins out of your body. And if you are constipated, consider some laxatives (such as prune juice) to avoid the toxins in your stool being released back in your system. Lastly, take chia seeds and anti-oxidants such as Vitamin C, to help get rid of the toxins.

It is important to take your time when you detox, as your body will struggle to process the toxins released from your cells. You are likely to feel worse, particularly tired, before you feel better. With that in mind, it is best to start a detox when you have a long weekend or short holiday, and can afford to rest a lot.

Also, do not starve yourself whilst detoxing; on the contrary, it is important to get a lot of nutrients, so eat well, as much as you need. Stay conscious about calories though!

Food allergies and Sensitivities:

Most people are familiar with what are known as "immediate response" allergies. Anything that brings an instant reaction, such as a rash or vomiting, is an immediate response allergy. Peanuts are well known for such a response.

What you may not know is that fatigue, stress or weight problems may also be associated with allergies. Many common ingredients in the foods we eat everyday may be a contributing factor to these and other health complaints. Some chronic health problems are also linked to food intolerance. Such problems are delayed-response allergies, so-called because reactions can take hours or even days to surface after certain foods have been consumed.

Symptoms of food allergies include, but are not limited to, eczema and skin rashes, weight problems, digestive problems, headaches and migraines, tiredness and fatigue, IBS (irritable bowel syndrome), sinus and asthma problems.

Some reactions are not immediate and it may take time to determine what the root cause of the problem is. Continuous symptoms, however, are often linked to our diet or environment. Other possibilities include a deficiency in certain vitamins or minerals, so see your physician and get some blood tests done if you suspect you might have a deficiency or food allergy.

Worst of all, sometimes people crave the very thing they are sensitive to, without realizing it! By the way, Dr Lustig's research shows that sugar has an addictive aspect: some foods act like drugs on your brain! The "no sugar" diets are good as many modern packaged foods are loaded with sugar and excess sugar is stored as body fat, so try and select only natural foods or packaged foods with less than 5% sugar per 100g. Be careful though, as low-sugar foods can have a lot of sweetener, which tricks your sweet tooth, or increase the amount of fat and therefore calories. So be wise, and check the caloric content as well!

Removing the main culprits:

The main ingredients associated with food sensitivities are gluten, wheat, dairy, yeast, sugar and eggs.

Although these are the main causes, anything can potentially be a problem: you can proceed by elimination, but that's quite slow and difficult to do, or do a lab test as mentioned earlier. To be sure of what you are allergic to, both Nutrition and Allergy testing and Vitamin and Mineral Deficiency testing are required.

As the main culprits behind food disorders are dairy and gluten, many modern diets recommended a dairy-free, gluten-free (DF GF) period of detox. They will be covered in more detail below.

At its most severe, gluten intolerance is better known as coeliac disease, a medical condition where no gluten-containing grain (chief of all, wheat) can be tolerated. It is usually with the sufferer for life.

At lower level, gluten sensitivity has been linked to a variety of modern ills, particularly related to brain and behavior disorders, because of gluten's potential impact on the gut.

Wheat sensitivity is easier to deal with, and in many cases can be eliminated through a strict elimination diet. Best to work with a clinical nutritionist so as to compensate any deficiency brought by the elimination of grains from the diet. The Western diet is high in wheat, it is used as a thickener in many prepared foods, so it is hard to avoid. Symptoms such as sinus problems, itching, fainting or dizzy spells, gastric problems, tiredness, rashes, and behavioural problems may be attributed to over-consumption of wheat.

Sugar sensitivity is on the increase, partly because of overuse, but also because there is so much hidden sugar in pre-prepared products, foods as well as drinks.

A large number of people are sensitive to yeast, and this is probably the hardest to deal with, as so many foods (and drinks) contain yeast. When combined with sugar and wheat overuse, a condition called Candida can develop, which can be very debilitating, resulting in tiredness, thrush, cystitis and other symptoms.

The last major food group is dairy, which consists of milk, butter, cheese, cream and yogurt, and a very large amount of children now have intolerance to dairy products.

None of these foods will affect everybody in the same way, though, so why you?

Well, each of us is dealt different cards are birth, through our DNA. But that's not the whole story: our food and environment plays a role too, by switching genes on or off. Epigenetics is a relatively new science, but the evidence is growing that the diet, sleep and exercise all play a role in our genetic response to the environment.

Let's now expand on the two most common food stressors:

<u>Going dairy free (DF)</u>:

Dairy can be an issue for several reasons, lactose being the most infamous. However there are other potential issues with dairy, such as casein.

Start completely dairy-free, in other words no milk, cheese, yogurt or any other dairy product from any animal milk (cow, sheep, goat and others). Use plant "milk", such as oats, coconut or almond milk; check the content though as cheap brands will have as little as 2% oat / coconut / almond and be nothing more than flavoured water. Also check for added sugars and any artificial additive.

My personal favorite is organic, no added-sugar, almond milk: it goes well with everything, including tea and coffee, and kids usually like it.

If dairy is your main source of calcium, consider a supplement, and balance it with magnesium. Some of the oat / coconut / almond milks available have added calcium options.

And include a probiotic in your diet.

After a couple of weeks, reintroduce dairy starting with cheese or (natural) yogurt from sheep or goat milk, and then milk itself. If that works for you, then you can try cow's milk, but check for any symptom: feeling bloated, constipated, any headache…

<u>Going gluten-free (GF)</u>: This is probably the most difficult part as such a big part of our modern diet contains wheat and other grains that have gluten. It is all the more difficult as many of the "gluten-free" alternatives usually contain high GI flours (rice, tapioca, etc.) that have a negative effect on blood sugar and waistlines!

So you will need to check the labels very carefully.

You can get buckwheat pasta (buckwheat is not related to wheat and doesn't contain gluten): they are not as tasty as the real thing, but with some nice tomato sauce, grated veggies and (organic) mince meat, you won't taste the difference. You can also get rice noodles, but check the labels for MSG and other additives.

Grains that are gluten-free and therefore ok: rice, amaranth, millet, quinoa and buckwheat.

For breaded product, best is to make it yourself: get almond meal instead of bread crumbs, roll in egg first, and here you go!

Breads are more difficult: choose corn tortillas or rice crackers if you can't live without bread. Add some fatty food (spread avocado or olive for instance) to balance the GI. Same for pizza: gluten-free options are widely available (but go easy on the cheese!).

Pastries will have to become a special treat, as there's really no place for them in a healthy diet. Keep them for special occasions.

The "GF-DF" recommendation is part of all diets aiming at reducing inflammations; it is worth trying.

If it helps and you feel better, keep the offending foods out of your diet.

4 – The "Really Simple" diet

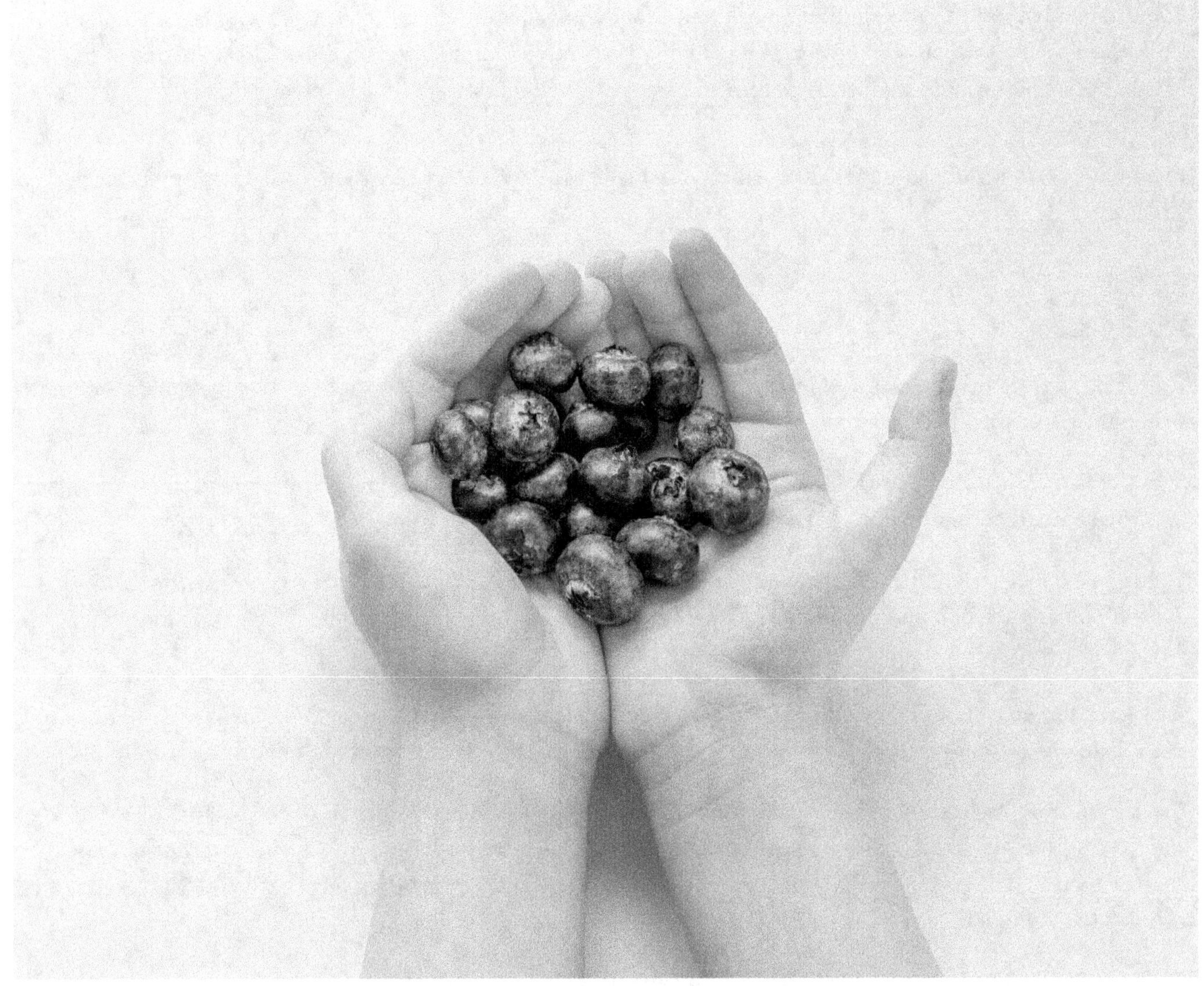

A healthy diet is about getting the right nutrients in the right amount and avoiding toxins as much as possible.

For this, a healthy digestion is paramount, and is as important as the quality and quantity of food ingested:

Healthy food supports the overall digestive process, which in turn helps extract more nutrients.

On the contrary, easting unhealthy food means the digestive process will get damaged: leaky guts, kidney or liver problems, IBS, and so on.

<u>**About digestion**</u>:

Healthy digestion is important: do you feel bloated? Constipated? As a guideline, make sure you get plenty of fiber (preferably from fruits and vegetables, or as a supplement such as psyllium husk). You can also improve digestion with the help of probiotics (choose a brand that has a good mix of strands and billions of each) and digestive enzymes.

If your digestive issue is severe, firstly seek help from a physician. Ask for food sensitivity tests, and enquire about the Specific Carbohydrate Diet. It is a highly restrictive diet, focused on a list of easy to digest foods. See if you feel better, and then start to reintroduce some of the restricted foods in your diet slowly, to check for any symptom.

If you have some reflux (sore throat, morning coughs, hoarse voice), try bicarbonate soda or apple cider vinegar.

About diets:

After looking at many diets and comparing common points and differences, there are really 2 main streams of thought regarding diets: plant-based and low-carb.

Vegan, Paleo, South Beach, Atkins, Dukan, Low GI, FODMAP, keto, alkaline… You name it, most diets end up in these 2 categories:

*Plant-based focuses on plentiful fruits and vegetables, low or no dairy, fish and egg, very low fat and no meat. If you are a vegan and completely avoid meat and eggs, you probably need a B12 supplement and maybe some iron.

*Low-carb focuses on, well, low carbohydrates, especially low starch and few complex carbs: little fruit, no grain, legumes or pulses, plenty of meat, eggs, fish and (good) fats such as nuts or olive and coconut oils.

Apart from these two types of generic diets, there also are plenty "personalized" diets, such as those based on your blood group, body type, astrological sign and other! I believe a personal diet is the best, but meaning one based on YOUR tests results, that balances YOUR caloric needs, avoids foods that make YOU sick and includes the supplements YOU require.

Unless you have test results, in which case you can adopt directly the relevant diet, we will take an approach that works for most people and can be used as your starting point:

1 - Based on nutri-genetic research, we will start with a low fat / low carb / DF-GF diet.

2 - We will then add back (good) fats to the diet, to low carb / DF-GF diet.

3 - Then add back some good carbs, to DF-GF diet.

4 - And lastly, reintroduce slowly dairy and grains to a Mediterranean diet.

Based upon your own genes and lifestyle, you might stop at any step; but all will follow the same order.

The "Mediterranean" diet is our ideal diet, coming out on top in terms of health effect in most research: it is a balanced diet which emphasizes healthy ingredients. It is especially good for heart health and digestion, as it contains good fats such as olives, avocados and salmon as well as plenty of fresh fruit and vegetable, herbs and spices, legumes, nuts and whole grains complemented with some yogurt and cheese and the occasional glass of red wine. It is not a plant-based diet as it includes meat, eggs, fish and dairy, but recommends the bulk of caloric intake through plants and just a little bit of meat.

To summarise the approach regarding the diet, here is a simple table showing what you can have at each stage:

Low fat / low carb / DF-GF diet	Low carb / DF-GF diet	DF-GF diet	Mediterranean diet
Lean meat, white fish, eggs, fruits and vegetables, black coffee and tea, herbal teas, honey, herbs and spices, plant-based "milks"	Keep	Keep	Keep
	Add back healthy fats: avocados, olive oil, coconut oil, nuts (not peanuts), dark chocolate (above 80%), oily fish (not tuna) and red meat. Do not deep-fry.	Keep	Keep
		Add back whole grains, apart from gluten-containing grains, and starches: rice, sweet potatoes. Also add back legumes, beans and pulses, soaked or sprouted	Keep
			Add back dairy (yogurt and cheese), preferably from goat and sheep milk. Add back gluten, but only as whole grains. Note: add one by one, slowly, checking for any

          Always consult a physician before starting a diet

			reaction.
			Add back the occasional glass of red wine

Adapt to your personal circumstances if needed, for instance avoid some fruits and vegetables in a FODMAP diet, or meat substitutes in a plant-based diet.

For example, I am personally on a low-carb DF diet because of my genetics, lifestyle and food sensitivities.

I make the odd exception here and there… which I usually regret!

<u>The common guidelines are summarized as</u>: ALWAYS

-Avoid processed foods, especially containing flour and additives such as colorants and preservatives.

-Avoid sugar and sweeteners: choose products that have less than 5% sugar overall, and use some (raw) honey instead or (the natural sweetener) stevia. This includes drinks.

-Avoid "bad" fats (trans-fats, saturated fats), but olive oil and coconut oil are ok in moderation, as well as nuts. Avocado and salmon are particularly good. Add some flax or chia seeds to increase your omega 3 intake. Try and have them a couple of times a week minimum, as most of us have too much omega 6 and not enough omega 3.

-Avoid all soft drinks and limit your consumption of alcohol: drink plenty of water and some (black) coffee or tea; alternatively, try kombucha. If you need milk for taste, I'd suggest almond mild (check the almond content % though: good brands put 10%, poor ones 2%…).

-Have plenty of vegetables, especially greens and particularly cruciferous (broccoli, cabbage, cauliflower, sprouts) every day. Be careful about nightshades if you have autoimmune diseases: avoid potatoes (replace them with sweet potatoes if possible, or try the Caroma variety which has a lower GI) and reduce aubergines (eggplants), peppers and tomatoes. Try and peel your veggies before consumption. Limit your fruits intake to one a day due to the sugar content and prefer high-nutrient fruits such as berries. Vegetables are alkaline and help balance meat and dairy acidity.

Note that ideally half of your plate should be vegetables, one third carb/starch (such as rice, potatoes, pasta or legumes) and the rest proteins. Note that they are nutrient-rich foods and that if you count 'macros" the calories from carbs and proteins will be nicely balanced. Drizzle a bit of olive oil or a couple of nuts or some cheese if you want to increase your fat intake (e.g. for a keto diet)

-Include herbs and spices to flavour your dishes; replace table salt with pink Himalayan salt.

-Have as much variety in your diet as possible (on a weekly basis), and try and buy organic whenever possible (especially if you eat the skin, such as berries, apples, etc.). For meat, get grass-fed organic. If you eat a lot of meat, you might need to balance the glutamates they contain by having GABA supplements.

When grocery shopping (food and personal care at least), check the ingredients AND the nutrition information on the packaging, particularly calories, as well as sugar content and type of fats.

A few other points, which are more specific to certain diets but good to know about:

-Do not mix proteins and starch: have your steak with a salad rather than potatoes, rice or bread. So no pies or ham sandwiches! The reason is that carbs and proteins are digested in different manners by the body, and mixing them slows down the digestive process.

-Lower your food GI by mixing any high GI food (e.g. white rice) with a low GI one (add some coconut oil for instance): cinnamon is a sweet spice that helps for any treat, such as popcorn.

-Once again, make sure you have plenty of veggies as they add fiber to your diet.

On-going weight management:

Coming back to weight loss, start your meal with protein and vegetables, then add a quantity of carbs and grains (such as rice or sweet potatoes) based on your level of physical activity and personal objectives.

If you want to lose weight, you should have very little carb apart from vegetables (which you can measure and track using apps such as MyFitnessPal).

Don't be a TOFI though! TOFI stands for "Thin Outside Fat Inside": people who eat very little, so don't look fat, but mainly eat bad things, so can actually have fat covering their organs (known as visceral fat) and health problems. Pay attention to what you eat, as much as to how much you eat.

*If you want to gain muscle, and are physically active (exercising intensively at least 30-45 minutes of exercise a day), you need to load your muscles: have a banana straight before exercise, to get some energy without a heavy stomach, and a mix of carb and protein immediately after exercise to bulk up and repair.

*For bodybuilding, you will need to eat a lot and often (every 2h). Body-builders will typically exercise for up to 4 hours a day and eat between 8'000 and 10'000 calories a day (3 to 4 times the maximum daily recommendation!). A body-builder's diet will be heavy in proteins, with some "good carbs" for loading (sweet potatoes and rice). Long-term, that could create problems for the kidneys, so we recommend drinking a lot of water and consider supplementing with GABA. Careful, some BCAA (amino acids) supplements can create problems for some people. We recommend to start with doing all your tests and check whether you can have a generic BCAA supplement or need to chose only specific amino acids.

Debunking Food Myths:

You probably hear of a lot of contradictory things about specific foods, so here is the laydown to help you:

-"Proteins is great":

The latest craze is added proteins. However, your body only need 7g of protein x kilogram of weight. Also, meat and dairy are strongly acidic, and the body regulates acidity by binding to calcium molecules coming from… your bones! So when having proteins, it's good to balance with vegetables, and maybe have some calcium chews (and magnesium) as well as GABA supplement to balance the glutamates.

Speaking about proteins, please reduce processed meats and small-goods such as bacon, sausages and ham: they contain nitrates as preservatives, which have been linked to higher cancer risks. Check if you can find nitrate-free brands instead.

-"Fat is fat is fat":

Not all fat are equal; some fats are good for health! If you struggle with fatty meals, you might have an issue with you gall bladder. That can be quite serious, so please get it checked. Taurine supplements can help; check with your physician. Good fats from olive oil, coconut oil, nuts, avocado, wild salmon are usually good for you, in moderation though: Fat (also know as lipids) is high in calories.

But more importantly, make sure you avoid the bad fats, especially trans-fats: avoid deep-fried dishes when eating out, as they sometimes use poor quality oil, and re-use again and again, turning it into a toxic brew! Yes, that means no fries, but you can have baked (sweet) potato chips instead.

-"I need sugar for energy!":

You might have heard your brain works on glucose, and so do your muscles… But that doesn't mean you need to ingest glucose or any other sugar! Glucose is actually manufactured in your body, so you can follow a ketogenic diet (high fat / low carb) and still feed your brain and muscles! Actually, good fats like Omega 3 are a great source of energy for the brain. The advantage of sugar is the rapid absorption in the blood stream, so if you feel tired mentally, eat a few grapes (the fruits with the higher source of glucose, rather than fructose) or have a banana before your exercise to replete your muscles' glycogen stores.

-"Super-foods are all I need":

Every year brings a new trend: from acai berries to kale to garcinia…

However most of these are not scientifically proven. What is proven is you need a variety of quality foods. If you feel like kale or berries, great; but do not expect any big difference to your health if that's all you do. To be honest, I think it's adding a level of complexity, so I would not worry or get out of my way to include the so-called "super-foods" in my diet. Best to have a balanced diet with all the common veggies!

If you want "super-foods", here are some of the unsung heroes:

Eggs, wild salmon, berries, green tea, avocado, olive oil, dark chocolate. Have these regularly, along green vegetables. Add chia seeds or spices such as cinnamon or turmeric to your dishes for flavor.

Remember, if we want to summarise this short guide in just one sentence, there's no secret ingredient, but the magic recipe is about balance: we need a mix of nutrients, and there's no absolute good or bad. There are bad fats and good fats, good carbs and bad carbs, good proteins and bad proteins. Choose more of the good and less of the bad ones, and you'll be on your way to a healthier you.

-"Whole grains are magic":

Whole grains are recommended in most diets, because of the fiber and extra nutrients you get. They also lower the GI of "white" grains, so are mainly beneficial.

However they can be harder to digest, and paradoxically the husk of the grain (also called bran or germ, ie the brown part) also contains some chemical compounds called lectins that can damage the gut lining. For that reason, paleo diets recommended to avoid ALL grains, including whole grains. We think if you limit your consumption and balance by having fruits and vegetables, then it is OK to include grains in your diet and that whole grains are healthier than refined grains.

So overall, better to have whole grain, but choose which grain you want carefully: rice, quinoa and buckwheat preferably to wheat for instance.

Make sure however that any "whole grain" food you buy is from complete grains, rather than added bran.

-"Raw is more natural":

There's been a trend, especially in the vegetarian / vegan diets, advocating for raw foods. Is it really better?

Well actually, you need a mix! Raw food will have more live enzymes and bacteria, whilst cooking usually extracts more nutrients. If you try and only eat raw food, which likely means a vegetarian diet with the occasional sushi and steak tartare, you are likely to be hungry all the time and get runny stools…

So, best is to have a salad as starter, with raw vegetables and sprouted nuts and legumes, followed by meat / fish / eggs with cooked vegetables. Once again, you don't need to balance every single meal, rather you need to balance your week: if you didn't have a salad today, try and have one tomorrow.

-"Organic or nothing?":

Ideally, choose organic whenever possible, particularly for meat/fish, eggs and dairy as they often contain added hormones and antibiotics. Regarding fruits and vegetables, if you can't afford or can't find organic, then don't worry too much: it's better to have them than reject them, but make sure you wash them.

-"Simple or Complex?":

Your body doesn't react the same way to all foods.

For instance, mono-saccharides are simple carbohydrate molecules that are easily digested and should be part of your diet, whilst di- and poly-saccharides are complex molecules that are harder to digest and might need to be eliminated if you have serious digestive issues. Only for digestive issues though: complex carbohydrates include beans and legumes, which give you gas, like beans and legumes as they are good prebiotic (they nourish your intestinal flora). To reduce gas, soak them overnight, or let them sprout first.

-"Fast or Eat every Hour?":

Very active people can eat 6 meals a day to keep fueling their body. But for most of us 3 meals a day are more than enough.

Actually, intermittent fasting can help to reboot your body, so if you're not sick or weak, by all means skip dinner from time to time. No evening snacking. Better yet: try an have an early dinner so you can have a "fasting period" from dinner to break-fast that is 10-12h.

-"Body part targeting":

Can you "shrink" one specific body part? Well, you will lose fat where your body accumulated it, so if you over-accumulate in your tummy, that's where you'll lose most. However one can't really "target" a body part for fat loss, but you can make it look better! Toning (through exercise) and massaging will help, especially regarding cellulite. But it's a cosmetic effect, not much more.

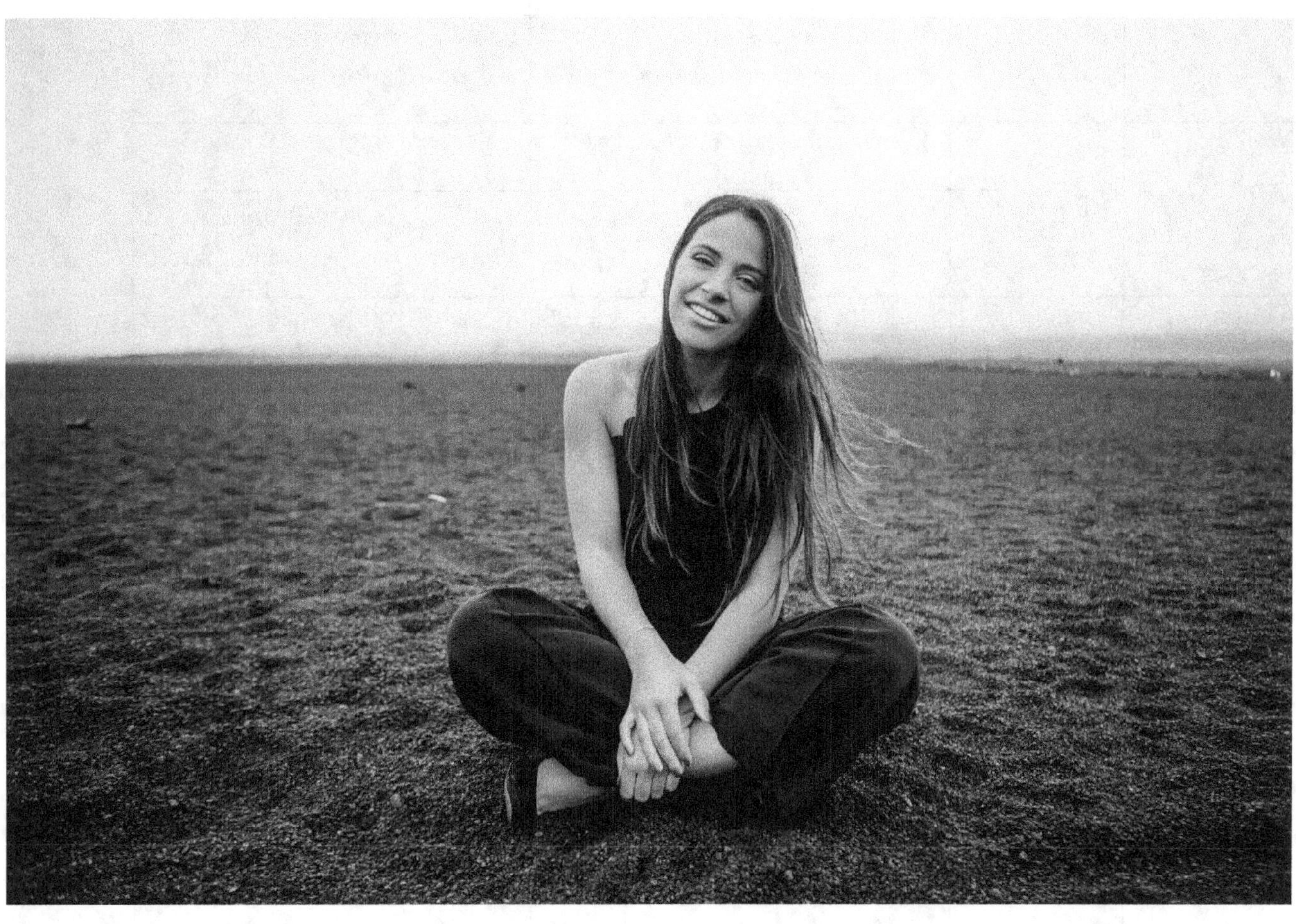

<u>Kick-starting the weight-loss process</u>:

The advice above is about long-term health and weight management, and it takes 3-4 weeks to change a habit (and taste-buds). That's partly why diets can be frustrating: nothing much happens in the first couple of weeks… But then the magic happens if you stick with it: the weight loss goes on automatic!

To help you with the first couple of weeks, here is an example of a simple menu inspired from the Mayo Clinic diet:

		Week 1	Week 2
Every day	Morning	1 grapefruit, 1 or 2 boiled eggs, black tea or coffee	black tea or coffee, 1 toast
Monday	Lunch	2 slices of ham, tomatoes, coffee or tea	2 eggs, spinach, tomatoes
	Dinner	1 toast, grapefruit, steak, salad, tea	Steak, salad
Tuesday	Lunch	2 eggs, 1 grapefruit	Steak, salad

	Dinner	Steak, tomatoes, lettuce, celeriac, olives, cucumber	2 eggs, 1 slice of ham, 1 natural yogurt
Wednesday	Lunch	2 eggs, spinach, tomatoes, tea	Celeriac, tomatoes, mandarin
	Dinner	Chicken, cottage cheese, cabbage, toast, tea.	Fruit salad, natural yogurt
Thursday	Lunch	Spinach, 1 slice ham, tomatoes	1 egg, carrots, a small piece of cheese
	Dinner	2 lamb cutlets, celeriac, cucumber, tomatoes	Fruit salad, natural yogurt
Friday	Lunch	Spinach, chicken, tea	Fish, tomatoes, carrots
	Dinner	Fish, salad, 1 toast, tea	Steak, fennel or celeriac
Saturday	Lunch	Fruit salad (any fruit, as much as you want)	Chicken, salad
	Dinner	Steak, cucumber, tomatoes, celeriac, tea	2 eggs, carrots
Sunday	Lunch	Chicken, tomatoes, grapefruits	Meat, fruits
	Dinner	Steak, cucumber, tomatoes, tea.	Whatever you wish, but in moderation!

Note that grapefruit can interfere with absorption of certain medications, so please check with your physician first.

It is not easy for the first few days due to the caloric restriction. However this diet works very well in rebooting your metabolism and kick-starting weight loss. But it is not a healthy diet long-tem, as it doesn't include many important foods. If it is too hard, increase the quantity but do not change the menu.

And remember, due to the detox effect, you might feel a bit tired and maybe have a headache or two: hang on, it's worth it!

It is also very easy from a groceries point of point, as the shopping list is limited. If needed, you can switch some ingredients around: for instance, if you do not like steaks, you can have more chicken or fish instead.

For the 2 weeks, please do not snack between meals. Only use a little bit of olive oil for cooking or seasoning salads and vegetables. No milk. No sugar or sweetener. No alcohol.

You will notice there are some foods otherwise not recommended, such as toasts. However the quantity is very limited and we believe balance is the most important.

After the 2 weeks, you'll need to decrease the number of eggs to a maximum of 1 or 2 per day. Yes eggs contain cholesterol, but mostly the "good" one, HDL. You can stop the grapefruits.

After the 2 weeks, you can also evolve your diet towards a Mediterranean one by adding back (olive) oil, low-sugar yogurts, and even the occasional glass of (red) wine! When happy with your weight, add back some whole grains, beans and pulses as well. Keep counting calories and checking for ingredients, types of fat and sugar level.

What you can't add back are the processed foods, sugary foods, flours and obviously anything you might be sensitive to.

About willpower:

Now, dieting is hard, so here is how to help your will power:

-Firstly, get rid of all "bad food" in your home, car and office! No exception!!! In other words, remove all temptation!

-Eat before you go get groceries, so you are less tempted to buy naughty stuff. Prepare a list, and stick to it.

-Always have some fruits and nuts at home, in the car, in the office, in your bag in case you're hungry and need to snack. Don't wait until you are starving as hunger drives us to the fast-releasing energy sources, which are usually sugary. Better to snack little and often, for instance some cottage cheese (if you're ok with dairy) with cinnamon and chia seeds, maybe some almond slivers or a few berries…

-Eat the same regularly, so you don't need to think about it! It's ok to have the same breakfast (e.g. a couple of boiled eggs) and snacks (e.g. the cottage cheese mentioned above) every day, and vary your lunch and dinner to some extent so you don't get bored. The repetitive aspect means you're more likely to stick to it, and that's one opportunity less to eat the wrong thing!

-When going out with friends, tell them you're on a diet (so they don't push you for the wrong food) and get a salad as a starter, meat or fish and veggies for main, fruit salad as dessert if you must, and yes, you can have a glass of wine and a coffee! If you eat more than 20% outside of your guidelines (in other words, you can have one "cheat meal" a week but no more), see if you can compensate by skipping dinner the following day (replace it by a can of tuna or some cottage cheese with a couple of veggies).

And what about supplements?

To be clear, you get much more from real food than from supplements: it's called bio-availability. However, if you are concerned your diet is not varied enough or your food not quality enough, then by all means get some supplements.

Be careful about provenance though, as some poor quality brands do not contain the promised ingredients. Worse, some can contain harmful ones, and damage your liver and kidneys!!!

Which supplements do you need?

Well, a couple are useful to all of us: magnesium, CoQ10, vitamin D for instance. Most multi-vitamins do not do much, so I'd suggest instead getting single ingredient if you can afford it. But best of all, you should be driven by test results: for instance, I have a methylation problem so I take methyl-B12, zinc, and a few other things that most people don't need extra of.

Note however you should check with a physician or clinical nutritionist as supplements can be tricky: for instance, cyano-cobalamine, a form of B12, contains a molecule of cyanide, which uses… B12! Some supplements can be toxic if taken at high dose or long term, such as B6 or selenium. Even vitamin C can give you loose stools if you have too much! And some other supplements need to be complemented for absorption (you need fat to absorb vitamin D) or to be balanced (chromium is needed when you take zinc, and magnesium with calcium).

Some supplements interact with absorption of medication, so always mention your supplements to your physicians.

Also, unless you are into bodybuilding, you do not need any protein supplement: the protein bars are nothing but snacks in disguise, and the powders usually contain dairy or soy. Even the protein powders made from rice or pea can be hard to digest, and not all BCAA (amino-acids) are good for you.

If you are worried about not eating enough proteins, just add an (organic) egg to your diet, including the yolk, or some legumes such as lentils if you are vegan.

Guts and digestion

Guts and the intestinal flora have become the main focus of digestive research recently, and some argue a link to the brain. The story goes like this: sugar and grains damage the guts, creating inflammation in the body and even sometimes leading to brain diseases such as Alzeihmer's.

Antibiotics and poor diet have reduced our intestinal diversity, and thereby hurt our first line of defense against bad bacteria.

To get your guts back on track, follow the diet guidelines below and make sure you take probiotics supplements daily. You can also include aloe vera juice and Manuka honey in your diet to help get rid of the bad bacteria.

One more important thing you might need to supplement if your stools are a bit hard: fibers!

<u>In summary: the Ideal Food Pyramid</u>

From this pyramid, make a list of your meals for the week, balancing proteins, carbs and fats over the week. Note this pyramid only contains the food you should eat, and excludes the foods you should not eat (such as processed foods!)

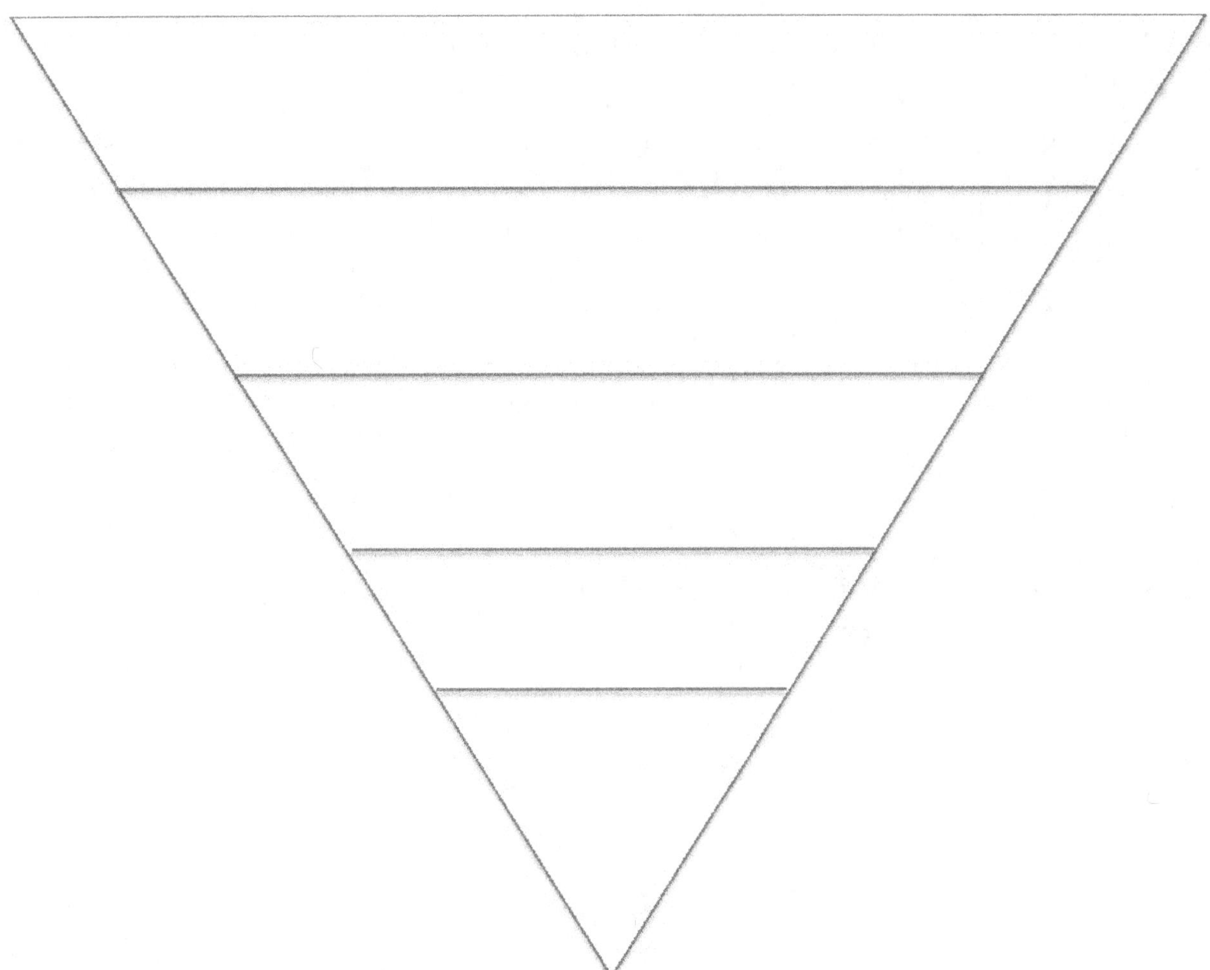

The pointy part at the bottom is what you can have weekly, and the large part at the top is what you can have daily. Don't forget to mix and get some variety!

Now, if you were expecting a whole bunch of recipes, there are none in this book, for a very simple reason: people don't follow the diet recipes for more than a few days… Too much hassle!
Instead, our approach is to start from your current meals and just make small tweaks to start with, changing your diet gradually rather than going cold turkey. This way, you have a better chance of sticking to it. And these changes will come from you discovering the caloric content and ingredients list of what you're eating, and deciding whether to keep as is, reduce, or stop and replace.

Keep it simple! Food your prepare should be simple (yet tasty), such as omelet with herbs, or salmon with salad. Fancy is good if you have time and love cooking, which is not true for most people…

There's no "miracle ingredient" we recommend, so you can use most of your existing recipes – just choose wisely: do the ratatouille rather than a pie, or replace your usual flour with almond flour! And make sure you put it all in your app, so you know how calorific your dinner is!

          Always consult a physician before starting a diet

<u>A few examples</u>:

For breakfast, have some eggs either boiled with ½ avocado or as an omelet with spinach.
Alternatively, have a natural sheep milk yogurt with organic berries, chia seeds and some cinnamon.
Or why not make a smoothie with spinach, berries, apple cuts and ½ banana, with some almond milk.
For kids who want cereal, try gluten-free, low sugar ones and add some raw honey if needed. Use a milk substitute if they are sensitive to dairy.

For snacks, a small piece of fruits, a few nuts (4-5, not more), and a piece or two of dark chocolate (80% at least, 90% preferably). Dark chocolate with nuts or fruits doesn't taste too bitter, and -after a couple of weeks getting used to it- your taste-buds will adapt.
If you are not in weight-loss mode, then dried peas, beans or corn can add some variety.

For lunch or dinner: mixed salad, meat or fish and some veggies. For salad sauce, make a vinaigrette with some olive oil, apple cider vinegar, herbes de Provence, mustard and Himalayan (pink) salt.
Make a chicken curry using coconut milk and turmeric, or mince meat with tomato sauce and some herbs.
You can have these with rice or quinoa for instance, but make sure you also add some veggies to the mix: courgettes (zucchini) and rice mix well for instance. Cook pumpkin or spinach in coconut milk or tomato sauce.
You don't need meat / fish at every meal: have some at lunch and not dinner, or vice versa.
By varying the spices and herbs you use, you can have the best of both worlds: a simple shopping list as well as some taste and variety so you don't get bored eating the same!
And make your life easy: fresh is best, but frozen is not far behind and can actually be better if snap-frozen. Just make sure in both cases you chose organic if possible.
Avoid canned and obviously packaged foods.

5 - Sleep

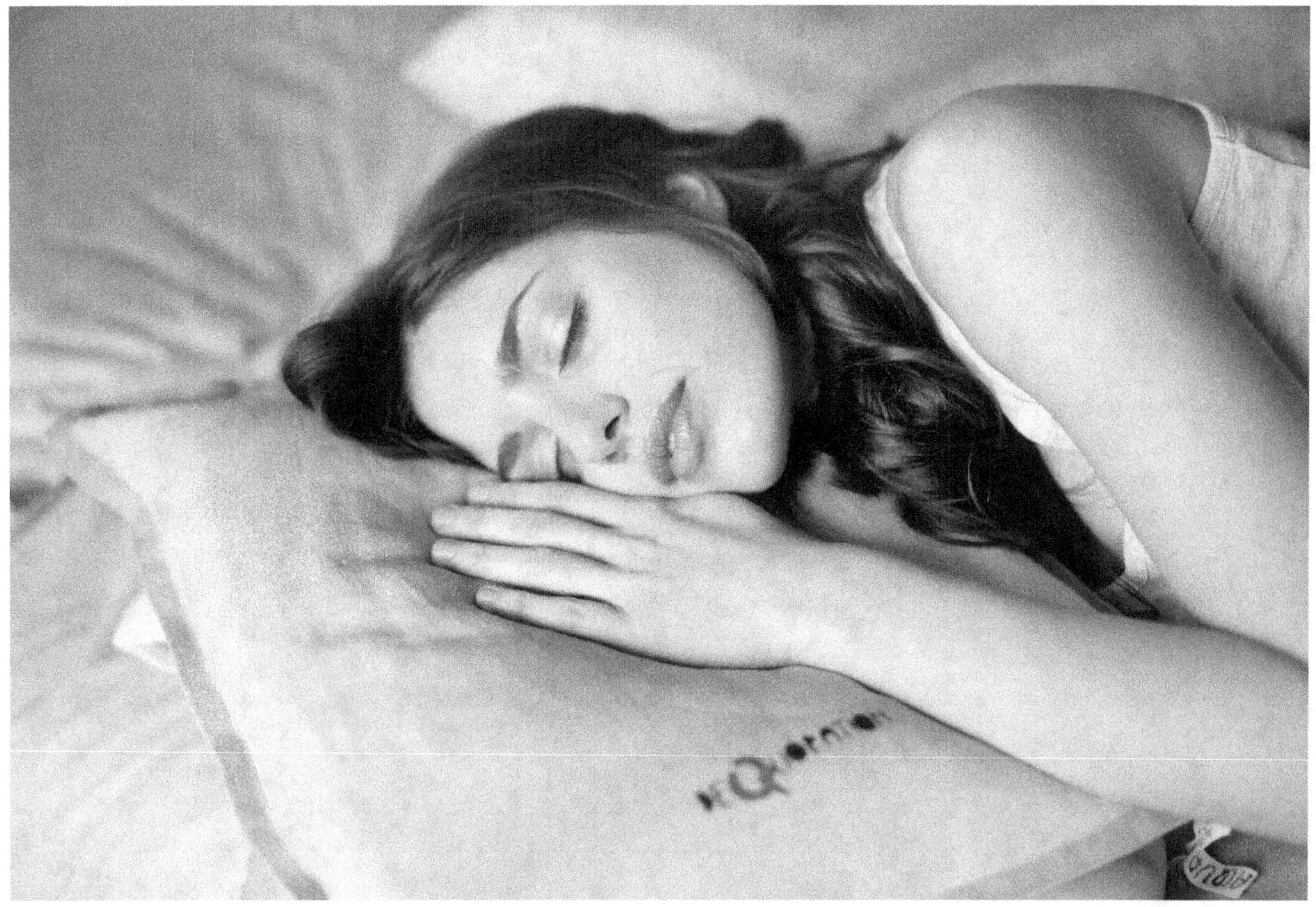

Sleep is a tricky topic. It sounds easy: just go to bed earlier and everything will be fine... Not so fast!

As per diet, sleep is about both quantity and quality. In the short term, a bad night means a bad day, feeling grumpy and tired. Over the long-term, deprivation is harmful. Sleep deprivation wreaks havoc with your hormones and your appetite control. When you feel tired, you have less self-control and crave for "naughty foods".

And you might not even know you're sleep-deprived! You can get used to the feelings, compensate with caffeine, or think you're ok because you went to bed early last night. But bad sleep accumulates like a sleep debt and one good night doesn't make it all go away.

How do you know beyond the "feeling tired" side? Other symptoms include "brain fog", in other words finding it difficult to focus and think, being grumpy, or feeling hungry...

Even if you go to bed relatively early, your sleep quality might be poor: a partner snoring or moving too much, a bedroom not dark or quiet enough, sleep apnea, reflux or any other condition might mean poor sleep.

You can go and get a "sleep study", which means a bunch of wires and a night in a specialized clinic to monitor your sleep quality. But before that I suggest getting a Fitbit or any other tracker that gives you an idea of whether you have a good or poor sleep quality. These trackers tell you whether you had an agitated (or restless) sleep or not, and give you an indication of your heart rate whilst sleeping.

If you want to sleep better, here are the guidelines

-Keep it dark and quiet! If needed, get new curtains, wear a mask, use earplugs, and maybe change your windows to double-glazing if noisy.

-Keep it cool: it's better to have a cool temperature and use a blanket.

-Get physical: exercising will make your body tired and help you sleep better. Also, sunlight will help regulate your melatonin and thereby your sleep cycle.

-Don't eat or drink for a couple of hours before bedtime. If you go to bed at 10pm, then try and finish your dinner by 8pm. If you want something after, have a herbal tea. Rooibos is naturally caffeine-free and tastes nice, but most herbal teas will do. Add some almond milk if you need, and some stevia or a spoonful of honey if you must.

-Relax: do not use phones or tablet in the 30' before going to bed as they emit a type of light that disturbs your melatonin production and keeps you awake. If you are worried about anything, try and meditate: focus on your breathing and on relaxing each part of your body one by one.

-Stick to a routine: go to bed at the same time every night, and go to bed early enough to have about 8h sleep. Ideally, you should be able to wake up naturally (so without the help of an alarm clock) at the right time. Keep your alarm clock just in case, but it should just be to listen to the morning news!

-Reset: if needed, to fall asleep more easily, try and have some melatonin. You need a physician script in some countries to get it. It's available over the counter in the US though, so speak to your chemist.

If you wake up naturally a bit earlier than your required time, start the day with some meditation or some stretches for a few minutes.

6 - Exercise

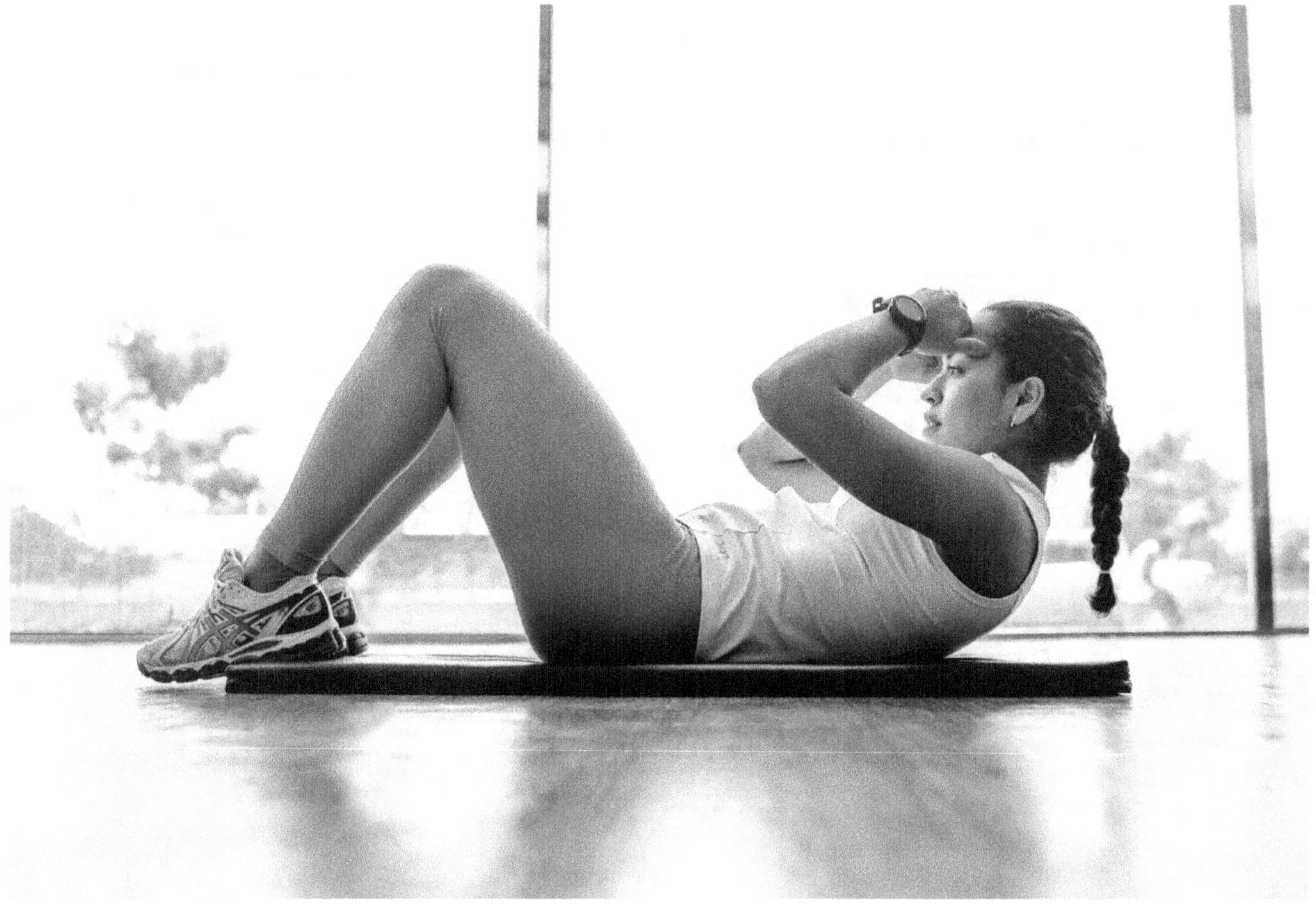

Exercise: you know you need it, but, hey, it's too hard! Not enough time, not enough energy…

Well, start slow: you'll be pleased to know you don't need a lot to reap some reward!

Firstly, try and go for 20' walks every day if you can. That's the bare minimum.

During weekends, either try and increase the pace a bit, or go for longer walks – up to 90'. The objective is to increase (slightly) you heart rate – don't go get a heart attack though!

When you've sorted your diet and sleep, doing some exercise will create a positive loop, helping with both better sleep and better weight management. Yes, it all works together.

If you can spare another 30' now and then, try and get some variation over the week between 3 types of exercises:

-Cardio: fast walk, hike, jog, swim, bike ride or even some soccer with the kids.

-Stretch and flexibility: yoga or pilates once a week – will also help with balance.

-Light weights: for muscular and bone density.

          Always consult a physician before starting a diet

You don't need a gym for any of this: do at home or outside. You don't even need any equipment: use your own body weight if you don't want to buy dumbbells! Push-ups, crunches, push-ups, squats, there's a lot you can do!

About HIIT – High Intensity Interval Training

HIIT is a burst of exercise at your highest intensity (so, as hard and fast as you can) for a short period, about 20 to 30 seconds. Think sprints.
If you are feeling well enough and do not have breathing or heart problems, including 2 or 3 HIIT bursts in your workouts will speed up your metabolism and thereby your weight loss.

Here is an example of weekly bodybuilding programme, which can be done at home. It will help tone your body, strengthen your muscles and bones. Most exercises do not require anything, apart from the ones with an asterisk: skip these ones if needed and repeat another exercise instead. For arms, shoulders and back, you will need a light weight: best to buy a pair of dumb-bells, otherwise use a heavy book or anything small enough for you to grab yet heavy and solid enough.

Start with a 5-minute warm up: slow "jog" moving your arms and head slowly at the same time.
If you have access to a gym, then go for rowing as it uses every muscle in the body!

Day 1	Legs	Squats, lunges, jumps, steps
Day 2	Core	Plank, side plank, crunches, abs wheel*
Day 3	Arms and shoulders	Dips (on chair or sofa), curls*, bridge
Day 4	Back	Deadlift*, chin-ups*, bended rows*, kettle-bell* swings
Day 5	Chest	Variety of push-ups (changing the width), bench-pressing*
Day 6	Cardio	Jog, swim* or ride bike*, skip rope* (at your own pace, for 30-45 minutes)
Day 7	Stretch	Slow stretch of every body part for 30 minutes

If you are not familiar with any of these exercises, you can check them out on YouTube or use of the many available free companion apps, such as Men's Health Workout Lite, Fitness Buddy or Fitness Pro.

Do as many repetitions of each exercise as you can, at least 4, then have a 30" rest, repeat for a total of 3 sets of each exercise. It should take 15 minutes overall, so total 20-25 minutes adding warm-up and cool-down.

If you are fit enough and do not have any heart condition, try and include 2 or 3 HIIT in between, to raise your heart rate and speed up your metabolism: for instance, do 30 seconds of star jumps or sprint.

End each session with 2 minutes of stretches to cool down, starting from your feet and going up your body, so as to reduce any soreness due to the lactic acid. Try a Magnesium supplement if you are getting cramps, or Epsom salts in your bath.

If you can't find the time every day, try to do at least 2 sessions during the week (and some cardio or stretching during the week-end), mixing one exercise from each body part and changing for each session (for instance, you might do squats for legs, plank for core, and push-ups one day, and lunges, crunches, bridge and different push-ups another day)

If you can manage both this session and a lunchtime walk, you'll be on your way to better health! And you'll soon see improvements… and results!

7 - Stress Management

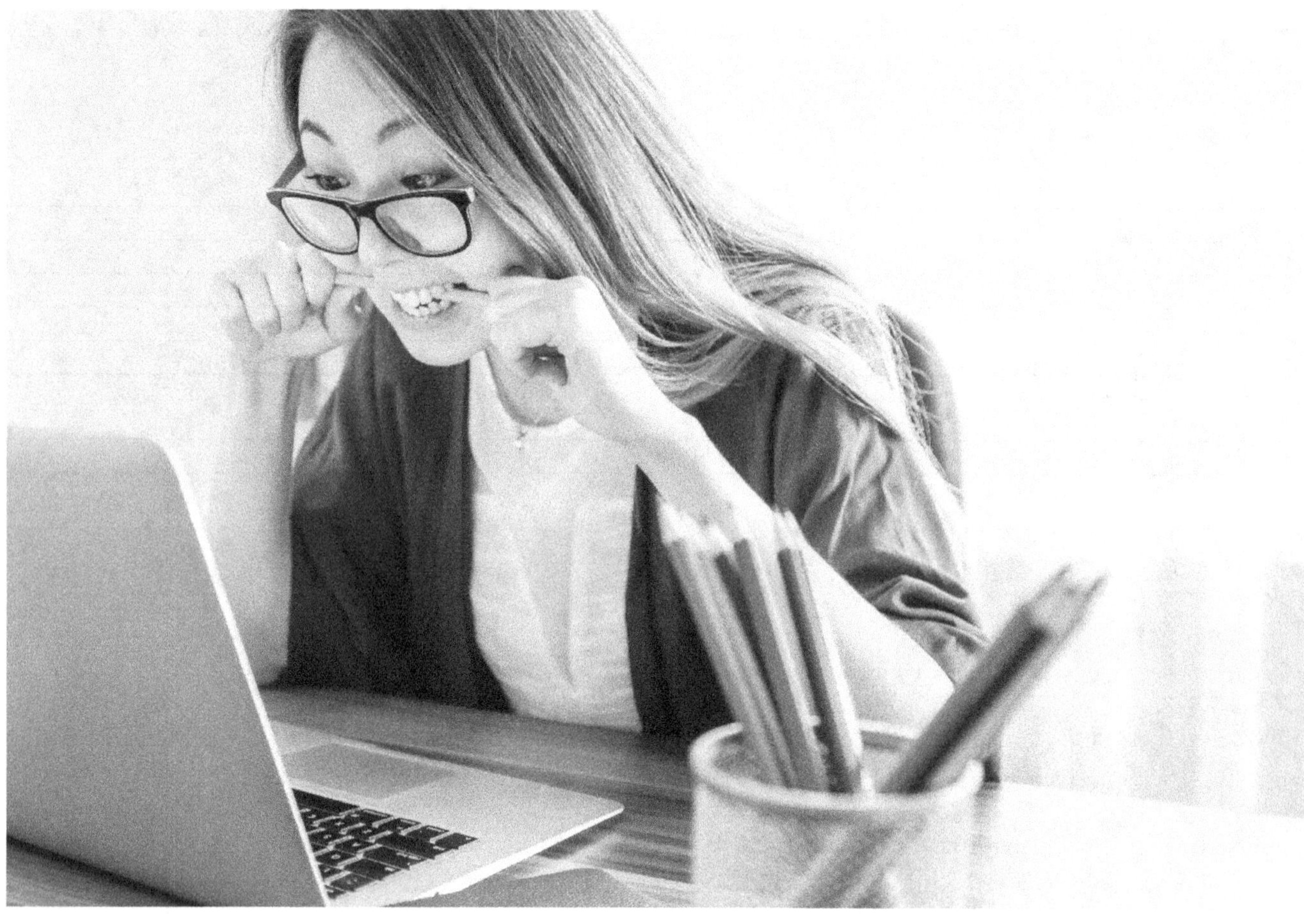

Stress is a plague of modern times. Everybody feels stress all the time. That's not healthy, as the "fight or flight" reaction puts our body under pressure.

Stress impacts our hormones, especially cortisol, our sleep and many other aspects of our health.

Worst is, it's usually hard to remove the source of stress. So we'll focus more on managing it than trying to get rid of it.

A healthy lifestyle helps reduce the consequences of daily stress: sleep, exercise, deep breathing and meditation all help and have been discussed earlier. Meditation, especially Mindfulness, is particularly recommended.

If you can, go for a walk or run in the morning rather than the evening: the morning sunlight is good for the mood.

A few other things you can do:

-Give yourself more time: if you get stressed about always running late, try and plan a bit more time. Set your alarm clock 10' early. Leave for school drop off or work 10' early. And so on.

-Get a diary and keep a personal journal, writing every day 3 good things that happened to you that day. Write in detail, so you can visualize the good times.

-Reduce caffeinated products, as caffeine increases cortisol, the stress hormone.

-Take a multi-B vitamins supplement.

-If you feel stress is getting out of control and leading towards depression, don't wait to burn out: get some professional help. Your can read about "positive psychology" (Martin Seligman) for some useful techniques.

8 - Variations

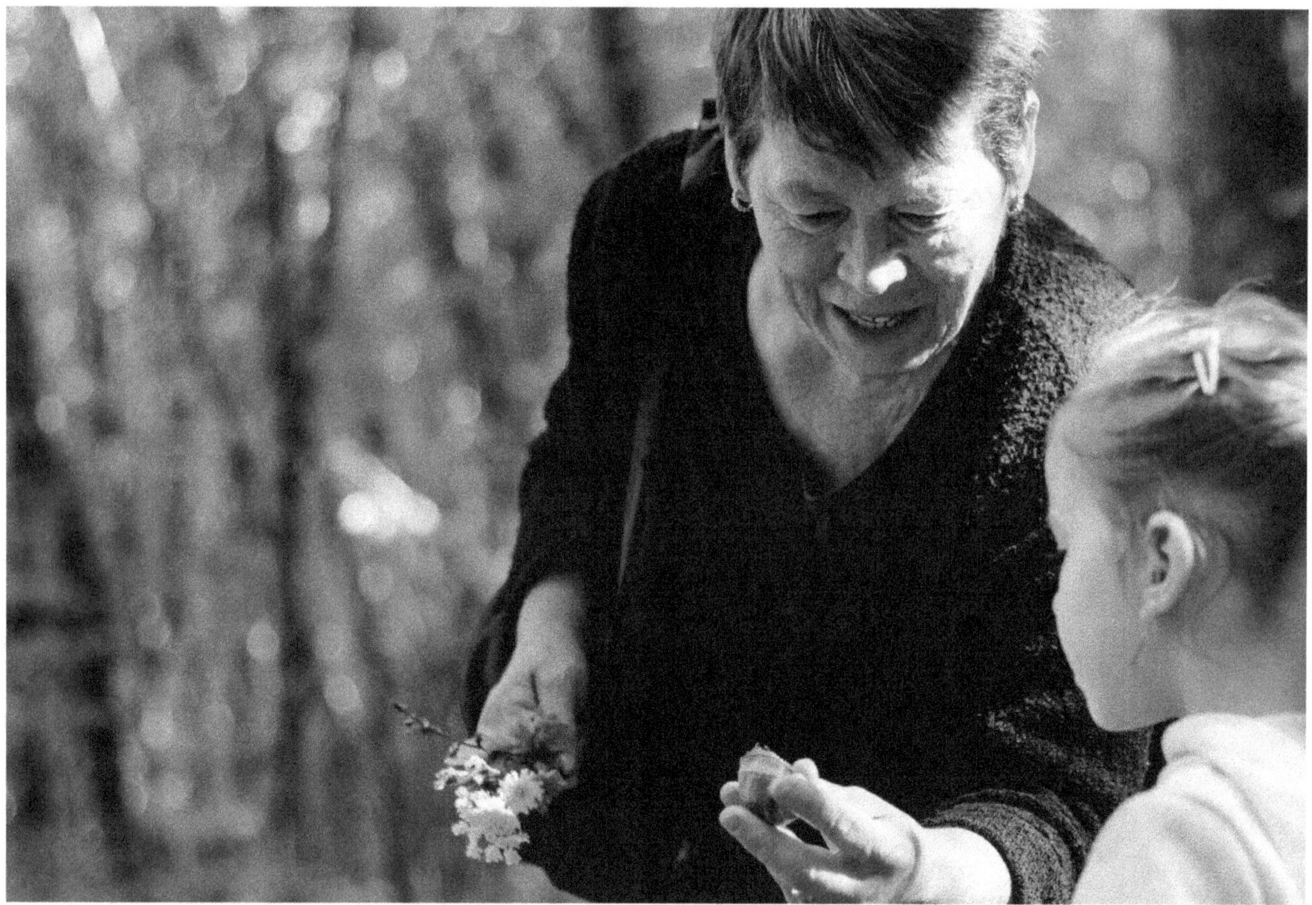

Not everybody is the same. This part tries to explain how to adapt the guidelines for specific people.

<u>For kids</u>: We do not recommend any restrictive diet, unless they have a diagnosed medical issue.

Kids need variety: they should have meat / eggs / fish and carbs such as fruits and vegetables.

Give them some grains, including bread and pasta, but prefer whole-grains and follow the guidelines for GI.

If they have any digestive issue, check for food sensitivity, but otherwise try and give them a varied diet as much as possible.

Let them eat as much or as little as they want, within the following guidelines:

-Reduce sugary foods (cereals, pastries) and sugary drinks (including soft drinks and juices).

-Reduce artificial flavourings, colourings and preservatives.

                Always consult a physician before starting a diet

-If you are worried about attention-deficit, make sure they sleep enough, reduce screen time, take them outdoors whenever possible and try and avoid gluten (from wheat and most other grains) for a couple of weeks.

-Give them probiotics – you can sprinkle them in yogurt or cereal if needed, as long as the food is cold: heat destroys probiotics.

<u>For pregnant women</u>: Follow the usual guidelines for pregnant women, especially folate (folic acid), but beware of most other supplements, as not all are safe for the baby. Definitely check with your physician.

Try and have a diverse diet, so the baby can have a broad range of nutrients.

Take probiotics.

The same is true whilst breast-feeding.

<u>For older people:</u>

Older people often have medical concerns, especially risks of diabetes, cholesterol, arthritis and the fear of brain degeneration such as Parkinson's or Alzeihmer's.

Take fish oil, anti-oxidants and probiotics, and try and reduce alcohol intake, sugary foods and drinks, and consider going gluten-free to see if your inflammations get better.

Be careful as some supplements might interact with medication – always check with your physician.

<u>Men vs Women:</u> The guidelines remain the same to a large extent.

Men are likely to eat more, especially more meat, and drink more. They might therefore have more need for GABA supplements.

Hormones are the other, obvious, big difference between genders: red meats will usually boost testosterone levels whilst soy contains phytoestrogens. To help regulate hormones naturally, best is –for both men and women- to lose weight (as fat stores hormones) and to avoid non-organic meat, eggs and dairy.

9 – Putting it together

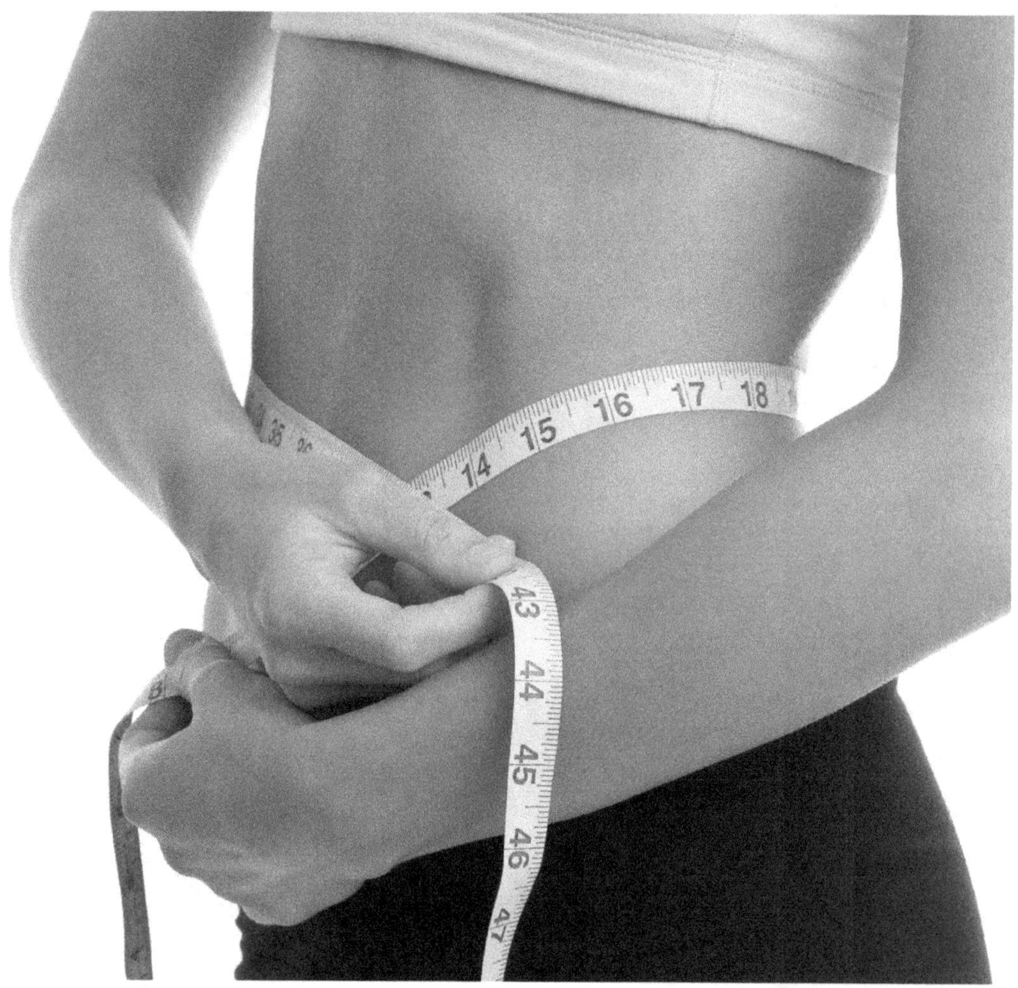

Congratulations on reading this short guide!

We hope it gave you clear guidelines on how to get your health back on track! And do not hesitate to get professional help from a physician.

Now what? You've read the guide and did some changes. Hopefully you're also seeing some results: feeling better, less tired, clearer skin, and a few kilos less…

How to keep the momentum? You need to keep track everyday to stay motivated: use a scale like Fitbit's Aria (that measures your body fat %), write a daily diary about how you are feeling, come back to this guide weekly to remind yourself of what to do and what not to do, and maybe read some of the other books mentioned below to understand the science behind the advice.

And to conclude, let's imagine you are catching up with a friend of yours over coffee…

You should be open and let people you are trying to get your health back on track. That will free you to choose the right dishes when eating out. And you will be getting a lot of support… and compliments!

                    Always consult a physician before starting a diet

When they ask about it, here is how you can explain:

The "Really Simple Diet" is more than a diet; it's a step by step method to a healthier life. Yes it includes diet and nutrition, but importantly is also deals with detoxification, sleep, and exercise.

It takes the learning from all famous diets out there and sorts out the useful, effective habits from the rest, to make it easy to understand and follow. Why read 50 books when you can learn as much from a simple guide? That's really what makes the Really Simple Diet method: it's useful yet easy!

Tell your friends to try it too!

We hope you liked this short guide.

In any case, please review it on Amazon and let us have your questions and comments on our Facebook page (@ShortHealthGuide): we'll make sure we update for the next edition. Thank you!

Further reading:

There are lots of documentaries on Netflix. Most of them dramatise the issues and add a lot of theatre. They make good entertainment but give you a skewed view, advocating a single "best" diet, providing only one side of the evidence.

If you want to read more, here are my top recommendations:

-Joseph Mercola, MD: Effortless Healing

-Patrick Holford: Improve your digestion

-Patrick Holford: Optimum Nutrition for the Mind

-Patrick Holford: The Optimum Nutrition Bible

-Gary Taubes: The case against sugar

-Gary Taubes: Why we get fat

-Dr Elisabeth Lipski: Digestive Wellness

-Prof Martin Seligman: Positive Psychology

-David Perlmutter, MD: Brain Maker

-David Perlmutter, MD: Grain Brain

-Dr David Lustig: Pure, White and Deadly: How sugar is killing us and what we can do to stop it.

-Mark Hyman, MD: The Blood Sugar Solution

-Gary E. Mullin, MD: The Gut Balance Revolution

-Joel Furhman, MD: Eat to Live

-Dean Ornish, MD: The Spectrum

-William David, MD: Wheat Belly

-Mark Williams: Mindfulness

-Tim Spector: Identically different

-Terry Wahls: The Wahls Protocol

-Justin & Erica Sonnenburg: Gut Reactions

Resources:

www.mindd.org

www.gapsdiet.com

www.dramyyasko.com

          Always consult a physician before starting a diet

www.ingramcontent.com/pod-product-compliance
Lightning Source LLC
Chambersburg PA
CBHW060521120726
48002CB00011B/3271